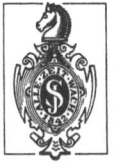

A.H.C. Ratliff · J.H. Dixon
P.A. Magnussen · S.K. Young

Selected References in Orthopaedic Trauma

Foreword by A. Graham Apley

Springer-Verlag
London Berlin Heidelberg New York
Paris Tokyo

A.H.C. Ratliff, ChM, FRCS
Emeritus Consultant Orthopaedic Surgeon,
United Bristol Hospitals, 2 Clifton Park,
Bristol BS8 3BS, UK.

J.H. Dixon, MA, MCh (Orth), FRCS (Ed)
Consultant Orthopaedic Surgeon,
Weston General Hospital, Grange Road,
Weston-Super-Mare, Avon BS23 4TQ, UK.

P.A. Magnussen, MSc (Orth), FRCS (Ed)
Senior Orthopaedic Registrar, Bristol Royal Infirmary,
Marlborough Street, Bristol BS2 8HW, UK.

S.K. Young, MA, FRCS (Ed)
Consultant Orthopaedic Surgeon, South Warwickshire Hospital,
Lakin Road, Warwick CV34 5BW, UK.

ISBN-13:978-3-540-19556-6   e-ISBN-13:978-1-4471-1695-0
DOI: 10.1007/978-1-4471-1695-0

British Library Cataloguing in Publication Data
Selected references in orthopaedic trauma.
    1. Man. Skeletal system.
    I. Ratliff, A.H.C. (Anthony H.C.), *1921–* 617'.1
    ISBN-13:978-3-540-19556-6

Library of Congress Cataloging-in-Publication Data
Selected references in orthopaedic trauma / A.H.C. Ratliff ... [et
    al.] ; foreword by A.G. Apley.
        p. cm.
    Includes bibliographies and index.
    ISBN-13:978-3-540-19556-6 (alk. paper)
    1. Orthopedics–Bibliography. 2. Traumatology–Bibliography.
    3. Fractures–Bibliography. I. Ratliff, A.H.C. [DNLM: 1. Orthopedics–
        bibliography. 2. Wounds and Injuries–bibliography. ZWE 168 S464]
    Z6667.08S47   1989 [RD732] 016.617'3–dc19

© Springer-Verlag Berlin Heidelberg 1989

Filmset by Fox Design, Surbiton, Surrey

2128/3916–543210 (Printed on acid-free paper)

Foreword

In medical writing brevity is the kiss of life. Nevertheless most articles are unnecessarily lengthy and publications continue to multiply. Pity the poor reader! A succession of unduly long articles is bad enough, but if each is followed by a plethora of references the effect is positively daunting. Even the reader who is impressed by the length of a list may question the author's discrimination. Were all those references needed? Were they helpful? Has the author really read every one? All too often we look in vain for evidence of selectivity.

Here lies the strength of this book. The authors have combed the literature and culled it ruthlessly, selecting just a few hand-picked references on every important aspect of orthopaedic trauma. They have ranged widely but chosen narrowly, and with a sense of balance. And having selected, they have also distilled, adding a brief and thoughtful commentary on each group of entries.

The four authors, of varying vintages, met at frequent intervals to discuss each section in turn and to debate the value of every inclusion. I can almost hear the cut and thrust as well-informed views were exchanged, and also the sighs of relief as differences were resolved. The authors compare their meetings with those of the Editorial Board of the JBJS; since these are a delightful mixture of conflict, entertainment and enlightenment, what a marvellous time they must have had.

The end product is not just a book, but a new kind of book. Not one to be read at length, but one to be taken off the shelf whenever a definite topic needs to be pursued by trainees or their teachers. It is a guide book to the vast treasury of original papers, new and seminal, old and classic – but all worth studying. You might have chosen differently. Why not try? You may not succeed but you will certainly become wiser. However, the authors have, in my view, made one serious mistake; orthopaedic surgeons everywhere will give them no peace until they produce a companion volume on cold orthopaedics. Please hurry.

March 1989   A. Graham Apley

Preface

It is astonishing with how little reading a doctor can practice medicine, but it is not astonishing how badly he may do it.
— Sir William Osler

Every young surgeon, having passed his Fellowship or Board Examinations and planning to become a consultant in traumatic and orthopaedic surgery, has gradually to learn to use the literature for his own personal sources of knowledge. Perhaps at times, he is bewildered by the enormity of the subject and the size of the journals. Standard textbooks will often list a large number of references at the end of each chapter, with no indication of their relative value. Our aim is to select a small number of authoritative references on important topics in orthopaedic trauma.

The book is a combined effort by four orthopaedic surgeons of differing age and experience. Two were senior registrars who were especially conscious of the needs of surgeons in training. Papers have been chosen on each subject after a weekly debate similar to that of an editorial board. Selection on some subjects has been difficult and no attempt has been made to include all important work. In this way, we hope we have kept the list of references to reasonable proportions.

The book is not intended to be a textbook. Articles have been included to present a balanced perspective on a subject and we have preferred those that are well written with a clear message. The larger chapters are those which we have found to be on controversial or rapidly changing topics and papers have been included to present both sides of an argument. If a subject does not appear to be topical or debatable and there are few publications, we have given it limited mention. We have tried to restrict sources of knowledge to easily obtainable journals but have occasionally included outstanding work in sources less easily obtained. We assume the reader has available some of the well known textbooks. Where indicated, we have selected impressive chapters in books, review articles or monographs on a highly specialised subject. Some classic articles have been included but only if knowledge expressed has stood the test of time.

Papers have been sub-grouped within each chapter to allow the reader to obtain rapid information on one aspect of the subject. After each group of references, a short commentary is given. The aims of this commentary are twofold. First, to indicate in one or two sentences why the named articles have been selected and second, to show the development and debate within a subject.

We hope this book will prove useful to the orthopaedic surgeon in training who needs to build up a core knowledge of the literature, and to prepare himself for the topical specialty Fellowship examinations. For the established orthopaedic surgeon it will provide a ready source of information to help with clinical problems as they arise.

Acknowledgements

We are grateful to all colleagues of the British Orthopaedic Association who have supported the theme of this book and have made many useful suggestions for references. Some have spent considerable time in advising the authors of their special knowledge.

The four authors would like to particularly express their thanks to Mrs. Penelope Bull who has done all the typing and production with great willingness and dedication. Without her tireless work, this book could not have been completed.

Bristol, 1989

A.H.C. Ratliff
J.H. Dixon
P.A. Magnussen
S.K. Young

Contents

Section 1: General Principles 1

The Multiply Injured Patient 2
    Incidence and Organisation of Treatment 2
    Assessment and Resuscitation 2
    Trauma Care Evaluation 2
    Problems of Management 3
    Massive Transfusion 4
    Fat Embolism 4
    Adult Respiratory Distress Syndrome 4
    Early Stabilisation 4
    Nutrition 4

Fracture Healing and Internal Fixation 6

Delayed Union, Non-Union and Bone Grafts 7
    Historical 7
    Basic Science 7
    Treatment 7
    Non-Union and Infection 7
    Operative Technique 7
    Electrical Stimulation 8
    Vascularised Grafts 9

Open Fractures 9

External Fixation of Fractures 10
    General Review 10
    Biomechanics 10
    Methods 10
    Complications 11
    Treatment of Non-Union 11
    Results 11

Pathological Fractures 11
    General Principles 11

Malignant Disease 12
Upper Limb Metastases 12
Lower Limb Metastases 12
Spinal Metastases 13
Myelomatosis 14
Paget's Disease 14
Osteoporosis and Fractures 15
Osteomalacia and Fractures 16
Stress Fractures 16
Pathological Fractures of the Hand 17

Vascular Injuries 17
Major Arterial 17
Compartment Syndromes 18
Volkmann's Contracture 19

Peripheral Nerve Injuries 20
General Review 20
Assessment 21
Surgery 21
Operative Technique 22
Reconstruction 22

Sudeck's Atrophy 23
The Classic 23
Clinical Studies 23

Paediatric Trauma: General Aspects 23
Basic Anatomy and Fracture Healing 23
The Growth Plate 24
Growth Changes in Long Bones 24
Remodelling 24
Principles of Management 24
Child Abuse 25

Tetanus and Gas Gangrene 26
Tetanus 26
Gas Gangrene 26

Section 2: The Upper Limb 27

Brachial Plexus Injuries 28
General Review 28
Investigation 28
Surgery 28
Follow-Up 28

Infraclavicular Injuries 28
Rehabilitation 28

Fractures of the Clavicle 29
The Classics 29
Surgical Treatment 29

Injuries of the Sternoclavicular Joint 30

Injuries of the Acromioclavicular Joint 30
Classification 30
Treatment 30

Dislocations of the Shoulder Joint 31
The Classic 31
Pre-Operative Assessment 31
Recurrent Anterior Dislocation 31
The Unreduced Dislocation 32
Posterior Dislocation 32
Nerve Injury 32

Acute Tears of the Rotator Cuff 33
The Classic 33
Treatment 33

Fractures of the Proximal Humerus 33
Classification 33
Treatment 34
Epiphyseal Injuries 34
Nerve Injury 34

Fractures of the Shaft of the Humerus 35
Clinical Studies and Treatment 35
Complications 35
Surgical Techniques 35

Fractures of the Distal Humerus in the Adult 36
Classification and Treatment 36

Supracondylar Fractures of the Humerus in Children 37
Remodelling 37
Methods of Treatment 37
Treatment of Cubitus Varus 38
Volkmann's Contracture 38

Epiphyseal Injuries in the Distal Humerus 39
Lateral Condyle.. 39
Medial Epicondyle 39

Dislocations of the Elbow 40

Fractures of the Radial Head in the Adult... 40
    The Classic.. 40
    Excision 40
    Internal Fixation 40
    Silastic Replacement 40

Fractures of the Head and Neck of the Radius in Children....................... 41

Fractures of the Olecranon 42

Fractures of the Shaft of the Radius and Ulna in the Adult 42
    Clinical Studies 42
    Surgical Technique 43

Fractures of the Shaft of the Radius and Ulna in Children 43
    Clinical Studies 43
    Volkmann's Contracture 44

Monteggia and Galeazzi Fractures 44
    The Classic.. 44
    Clinical Studies 44

Colles' Fracture... 45
    The Classic.. 45
    Conservative Treatment 45
    Surgical Treatment 46
    Complications 46

Smith's Fracture 47
    Clinical Studies 47
    Surgical Technique 47

Section 3: The Hand 49

Primary Treatment of the Acutely Injured Hand 50
    The Classic.. 50
    Primary Treatment 50
    Skin Cover 50

Anaesthesia in Hand Surgery 51

Fractures of the Scaphoid 52
    The Classic.. 52
    Natural History and Conservative Management 52

Non-Union 52
Surgical Treatment 52

Dislocations of the Carpus 53

Carpal Instability 53

Fractures of the Hand 54
Review Article 54
Bennett's Fracture 54
Fractures of the Metacarpals 54
Fractures of the Phalanges 55
Operative Technique 55

Dislocations and Ligament Injuries in the Digits 56
The Proximal Interphalangeal Joint 56
The Thumb Metacarpophalangeal Joint 56

Flexor Tendon Injuries 57
Historical Review 57
Biology 57
Clinical Aspects 58
Operative Technique 58
Tendon Grafting 58
Review Article 58

Extensor Tendon Injuries 59
Mallet Finger 59
The Boutonnière Deformity 60
Rupture of the Extensor Pollicis Longus Tendon 60
Operative Technique 60
Review Article 60

Nerve Injuries in the Hand 60

Finger Tip Injuries and Amputations 61
Clinical Studies 61
Amputations of the Thumb 62
Operative Technique 62

High Pressure Injection Injuries 63

Infections in the Hand 63
Clinical Studies 63
Specific Problems 63
Operative Technique 64

Replantation 64

Rehabilitation 65

Section 4: The Spine 67

Classification and Mechanisms of Injury 68

Spinal Cord Injury 68

Injuries of the Cervical Spine 69
    Clinical Studies and Pathology (C3–C7) 69
    Treatment (C3–C7) 70
    Hyperextension Injuries 71
    Fractures of the Odontoid 71
    Hangman's Fracture 72
    Cervical Instability 72
    Cervical Spine Injuries in Children 73
    The Paralysed Upper Limb 73

Injuries of the Thoracolumbar Spine 74
    Radiology 74
    Treatment 74

Fractures of the Pelvis 76
    The Classic 76
    Pathological Anatomy 76
    Clinical Studies 76
    Bladder and Urethra 77

Section 5: The Lower Limb 79

Dislocations of the Hip and Fractures of the Acetabulum 80
    The Classic 80
    Long-Term Results 80
    Management 80
    Review Article 81

Hip Fractures in the Elderly 82
    Historical 82
    Basic Science 82
    Epidemiology 82
    Osteoporosis and Osteomalacia 83
    Mortality 83

Sub-capital Fractures 84
    The Classics 84

Treatment 84
Avascular Necrosis 85
Stress Fractures 86

Inter-Trochanteric Fractures 86
The Classic 86
Epidemiology and Biomechanics 86
Complications 87
Treatment 87

Hip Fractures in Children 88

Fractures of the Shaft of the Femur 88
Conservative Treatment 88
Cast Bracing 88
Intramedullary Nailing 89
External Fixation 90
In Children 90
With Associated Injuries 91
Complicating Total Hip Replacement 92

Supracondylar Fractures of the Femur in the Adult ... 92

Supracondylar Fractures of the Femur in the Child ... 93

Soft Tissue Injuries of the Knee 94
Anatomy and Biomechanics 94
Assessment 94
Injuries of the Meniscus 95
Acute Ligament Injuries 95
Chronic Instability 97

Dislocations of the Knee 97
Conservative Treatment 97
Operative Treatment 97

Fractures of the Patella 98
Excision 98
Treatment of Comminuted Fracture 98
Technique of Fixation 98

Dislocations of the Patella 98
Acute 98
Recurrent 98
Habitual 99

Dislocation of the Proximal Tibiofibular Joint 100

Fractures of the Tibial Plateau 100
    Conservative Treatment 100
    Operative Treatment 100
    Review Article 100

Fractures of the Tibia 101
    The Classics 101
    Cast Bracing 101
    Internal Fixation: Plating 102
    Internal Fixation: Intramedullary Nailing 102
    External Fixation and Open Fractures 102
    Non-Union 103
    Ipsi-lateral Fractures of the Tibia and Femur 104
    Review Article 104

Ankle Fractures 104
    Classification 104
    Surgical Treatment 105
    Fractures in the Elderly 105
    Comparison of Operative and Conservative Treatment 105
    Long-Term Follow-Up 105
    Tri-Plane Fractures 105
    Review Article 105

Injuries of the Lateral Ligament of the Ankle 106

Rupture of the Achilles Tendon 107

Fractures of the Talus 108
    The Classic 108
    Biomechanics 108
    Blood Supply 108
    Classification and Operative Treatment 108
    Long-Term Results 108

Sub-Talar Dislocation of the Foot 109

Fractures of the Calcaneum 109
    The Classic 109
    An Atlas 110
    Radiology 110
    Treatment 110

Mid-Tarsal Injuries 111

Tarso-Metatarsal Injuries 111
    The Classic 111
    Classification and Treatment 111

Author Index 113

Subject Index 121

Section 1
General Principles

The Multiply Injured Patient

Incidence and Organisation of Treatment

Hoffman E **Mortality and morbidity following road accidents** Ann R Coll Surg Engl 1976;58:233–240

Trunkey DD **Presidential address: On the nature of things that go bang in the night** Surgery 1982;92:123–132

Anderson ID, Woodford M, De Dombal FT, Irving M **Retrospective study of one thousand deaths from injury in England and Wales** Br Med J 1988;296:1305–1308

Fischer RP, Flynn TC, Miller PW, Duke JH **Urban helicopter response to the scene of injury** J Trauma 1984;24:946–950

The management of patients with major injuries: report of a Working Party Royal College of Surgeons of England Commission on Provision of Surgical Services 1988

Assessment and Resuscitation

Harviel JD, Champion HJ **Early assessment of the acutely injured patient** Curr Orthop 1988;2:99–103

Thal ER, Raess DH **Early recognition and treatment of shock.** In: Myers MH ed. The multiply injured patient with complex fractures Philadelphia: Lea and Febiger, 1984;32–41

Trauma Care Evaluation

Baker SP, O'Neill B, Haddon W Jr, Long WB **The injury severity score – a method for describing patients with multiple injuries and evaluating emergency care** J Trauma 1974;14:187–196

Boyd CR, Tolson MA, Copes WS **Evaluating trauma care: The TRISS method** J Trauma 1987;27:370–378

In the United States trauma is the leading cause of death of people who are less than 44 years old and accounts for more than 150,000 deaths each year. **Hoffman** in 1976 described in detail the extent of the mortality and morbidity that results from road traffic accidents in this country. A prospective study on 344 deaths and 2392 surviving admissions collected over a one year period from twelve hospitals in the north of England showed a situation very similar to that in the United States.

In the USA **Trunkey** has shown a significant difference in outcome in the management of the severely injured, depending on whether patients were taken to the nearest departments offering an emergency service, or to a single specialised trauma unit. In the latter only 1% of deaths were considered to have been preventable whereas in the other, between 28% and 73% of deaths were considered preventable. It has now become accepted in the United States that the management of the severely injured should be concentrated in suitably staffed and equipped centres.

Anderson has recently published a retrospective study of 1000 deaths from injury in England and Wales. The results closely parallel those from similar studies in America and suggest there are serious deficiencies in the services for managing severe injuries in this country.

During 1981 the use of a helicopter service to the scene of injury in Houston was described by **Fischer**. In a large congested city with a poor freeway system, a valuable medical service was provided.

A **Working Party** of the Royal College of Surgeons has recently reviewed the results of two prospective studies concerning the management of major injuries in the United Kingdom. Major life threatening injury is rare but when it occurs, its management is imperfect. Detailed recommendations have been presented in this report, the major one being that the management of the multiply injured patient should be undertaken in suitably situated hospitals that can provide the necessary wide range of supporting staff, services and experience. It is suggested that a number of consultant surgeons should be encouraged to take a major interest in accident surgery.

Harviel has stressed that the initial hour in the care of the victim is the critical time for life and limb salvage. He described the rapid assessment of airway and circulation and discussed the use of basic fluid for resuscitation in the acute phase. The evaluation and treatment of the hypotensive patient, with a concise review of the different types of shock, is described by **Thal**. A borderline blood pressure (100–110 mm Hg) is often an early warning sign of impending disaster.

The problem of summarising assessment of injury severity was developed by **Baker** and was especially concerned with the patient with multiple trauma. The aim was to compare the mortality experience of varied groups of trauma patients and thus improve the care of the injured. This was further developed by the concept of TRISS and was discussed by **Boyd**. The cumulative effect of injury to several body systems was calculated and the resulting trauma score related to probability of survival.

Problems of Management

Heyworth J, Yates DW **Management of the severely injured patient** Surgery 1988;57:1351–1359

Bone L, Bucholz R **Current concepts review: The management of fractures in the patient with multiple trauma** J Bone Joint Surg [Am] 1986;68-A:945–949

Massive Transfusion

Riska EB, Bostman O, von Bonsdorff H, Hakkinen S, Jaroma H, Kiviluoto O, Paavilainen T **Outcome of closed injuries exceeding 20-unit blood transfusion need** Injury 1988;19:273–276

Fat Embolism

Peltier LF **Fat embolism – an appraisal of the problem** Clin Orthop 1984;187:3–17

Sevitt S **Fat embolism** London: Butterworth, 1962

Gossling HR, Ellison LH, De Graff AC **Fat embolism – the role of respiratory failure and its treatment** J Bone Joint Surg [Am] 1974;56-A:1327–1337

Gurd AR, Wilson RI **The fat embolism syndrome** J Bone Joint Surg [Br] 1974; 56-B:408–416

Lindeque BGP, Schoeman HS, Dommisse GF, Boeyens MC, Vlok AL **Fat embolism and the fat embolism syndrome – a double blind therapeutic study** J Bone Joint Surg [Br] 1987;69-B:128–131

Adult Respiratory Distress Syndrome

Weigelt JA **The adult respiratory distress syndrome.** In: Myers MH ed. The multiply injured patient with complex fractures Philadelphia:Lea and Febiger, 1984:42–54

Pepe PE, Potkin RT, Reus DH, Hudson LD, Carrico CJ **Clinical predictors of the adult respiratory distress syndrome** Am J Surg 1982;144:124–130

Early Stabilisation

Riska EB, Von Bonsdorff H, Hakkinen S, Jaroma H, Kiviluoto O, Paavilainen T **The prevention of fat embolism by early internal fixation of fractures in patients with multiple injuries** Injury 1976;8:110–116

Goris RJA, Gimbrere JSF, Van Niekerk JLM, Schoots FJ, Booy LHD **Early osteosynthesis and prophylactic mechanical ventilation in the multi-trauma patient** J Trauma 22;1982:895–903

Johnson KD, Cadambi A, Seibert GB **Incidence of adult respiratory distress syndrome in patients with multiple musculo-skeletal injuries: effect of early operative stabilisation of fractures** J Trauma 25;1985:375–383

Nutrition

Grant JP **Nutrition in the trauma patient.** In: Moylan JA ed. Trauma Surgery Philadelphia: JB Lippincott, 1988:501–533

Pre-hospital and early hospital management is described briefly and clearly by **Heyworth**. Problems of inadequate ventilation are outlined with their management. The controversy concerning the types of fluid replacement for hypovolaemic shock and the choice of fluid – crystalloid or colloid – is discussed. Most departments in the UK use colloid but the debate continues. A concise recent review of trends in the management of the multiply injured patient is provided by **Bone**. Compelling arguments are marshalled for the early fixation of fractures, not only to improve function but also to reduce the incidence of the adult respiratory distress syndrome and fat embolism.

Riska has discussed the outcome of closed injuries where massive blood transfusion had been required. A series of 129 patients with closed injuries receiving more than 20 units was analysed. Stored whole blood was the main replacement having previously initiated fluid replacement with crystalloid solutions. Mortality was high (25%) where the patients received up to 39 blood units. The syndrome of multiple organ failure is discussed.

The classic contributions by both **Peltier** and **Sevitt** on fat embolism have been included. **Gossling** has discussed the controversial subject of the pathophysiology of fat embolism. **Gurd**, in 1974, stressed the distinction which must be made between the fat embolism syndrome, a clinical entity, and fat embolism demonstrated pathologically which may be found after death. The clinical presentation of 100 cases of the syndrome are described and 16 of the patients died. **Lindeque** has recently reported the results of a therapeutic study and has suggested that methylprednisolone is effective in treating and reducing the risk of the fat embolism syndrome.

It is now considered essential to maintain arterial oxygen levels. The adult respiratory distress syndrome (ARDS) is the most severe pulmonary complication that can follow multiple trauma. **Weigelt** has defined the condition and summarised the incidence, morbidity, pathology and treatment. Although rare, mortality may be as high as 50%–70%. Aggressive cardiovascular monitoring and treatment is essential. **Pepe** described the incidence in a prospective study of 136 patients. There was a wide range of general problems, such as the sepsis syndrome, pulmonary contusion, multiple emergency transfusions and multiple fractures from which ARDS may develop.

On a study of a large number of patients, **Riska** has concluded that the incidence and clinical severity of fat embolism syndrome can be lessened in patients with multiple trauma by the early stabilisation of fractures of a long bone. **Goris** carried out a retrospective study of 58 consecutive trauma patients with multiple major injuries; early primary fixation of unstable fractures with aggressive ventilatory support prevented or attenuated the clinical manifestations of ARDS. **Johnson** has more recently confirmed these observations based on a study of 132 consecutive patients with a high index severity score. There was a significant increase in the incidence of ARDS associated with delay in operative stabilisation of major fractures.

Grant has produced a useful reference chapter on nutrition in the trauma patient including long-term fluid, carbohydrate and fat requirements.

Fracture Healing and Internal Fixation

Charnley J **The nature of fracture repair** In: The closed treatment of common fractures 3rd edn Edinburgh: E & S Livingstone, 1961:3–42

McKibbin B **The biology of fracture healing in long bones** J Bone Joint Surg [Br] 1978;60-B:150–162

Olerud S, Karlstrom G **Rigid internal fixation in fracture healing** In: McKibbin B, ed. Recent advances in orthopaedics 3 Edinburgh; Churchill Livingstone, 1979:163–174

Muller ME, Allgower M, Schneider R, Willenegger H **Aims and fundamental principles of the AO method** In: Manual of internal fixation, 2nd edn Berlin, etc; Springer-Verlag, 1979:3–27

Pahud B, Vasey H **Delayed internal fixation of femoral shaft fractures – Is there an advantage? A Review of 320 fractures** J Bone Joint Surg [Br] 1987, 69-B:391–394

The first chapter in **Charnley**'s book contains a thoughtful section on fracture repair. The union of cancellous and cortical bone, the function of the periosteum and the role of fixation in fracture union are discussed. Charnley considered that compression has a beneficial action on the union of cancellous bone but not of cortical bone. A provocative debate is presented on the pros and cons of the operative treatment of fractures. **McKibbin** summarised the healing process of a fracture and debated the clinical implications of external callus and primary bone union. **Olerud** produced a concise chapter on rigid internal fixation in fracture healing. The various types of this fixation have proved to be excellent aids in the practical management of fractures and pseudarthroses. The indications and contra-indications of the different techniques in various fractures are discussed. The aims and principles of the AO method are outlined by **Muller**. Bone reaction to compression, movement, and metallic implants is outlined. Compression greatly enhances the rigidity of internal fixation and it is considered that the strength of fixation should be such that movement is eliminated. The timing of internal fixation has recently been discussed by **Pahud** based on a study of 320 fractures of the femur. Contrary to a belief previously held by some surgeons, it was concluded that fractures do not unite more readily if fixation is delayed.

Delayed Union, Non-Union and Bone Grafts

Historical

Nicoll EA **The treatment of gaps in long bones by cancellous insert grafts** J Bone Joint Surg [Br] 1956;38-B:70–82

Basic Science

Friedlaender GE **Current concepts review. Bone grafts: the basic science rationale for clinical applications** J Bone Joint Surg [Am] 1987;69-A:786–790

Treatment

Muller ME, Allgower M, Schneider R, Willenegger H **Delayed Union and Pseudarthroses.** In: Manual of Internal Fixation. 2nd edn Berlin, etc: Springer-Verlag, 1979:334–355

Rosen H **Compression treatment of long bone pseudarthroses** Clin Orthop 1979:138;154–166

Shelton WR, Sage FP **Modified Nicoll-graft treatment of gap non-unions in the upper extremity** J Bone Joint Surg [Am] 1981;63-A:226–231

Non-Union and Infection

Oliveira JC de **Bone grafts and chronic osteomyelitis** J Bone Joint Surg [Br] 1971;53-B:672–683

Meyer S, Weiland AJ, Willenegger H **The treatment of infected non-union of fractures of long bones – a study of sixty-four cases with a five to twenty-one year follow-up** J Bone Joint Surg [Am] 1975;57-A:836–842

Kelly PJ **Chronic osteomyelitis in adults.** In: McKibbin B, ed. Recent advances in orthopaedics 4 Edinburgh: Churchill Livingstone, 1983:119–129

Burny F, Rasquin C **The "Papineau technique" using Hoffmann external fixation** In: Ackroyd CE, O'Connor BT, de Bruyn PF, ed. The severely injured limb Edinburgh, etc: Churchill Livingstone, 1983: 241–249

Operative Technique

Chapman MW **Bone Grafting.** In: Chapman MW, ed. Operative orthopaedics. Vol.1. Philadelphia: JB Lippincott, 1988:97–106

Nicoll described the bridging of gaps in long bones by the use of blocks of iliac graft and fixation with a plate. The operative technique of donor grafting from the ilium is illustrated with colour photographs.

Friedlaender discussed the various types of bone graft, their behaviour and factors influencing this behaviour. Cancellous and cortical grafts differ in the rate of repair.

The nature of hypertrophic and atrophic non-union are described by **Muller** and the principles of treatment summarised. He discussed how to treat non-union in the presence of deformity and infection. A 92% success rate in 122 cases of non-union treated by compression was reported by **Rosen**. In hypertrophic non-union, half the cases were successful without bone grafts and without dissecting the pseudarthroses. **Shelton** has updated Nicoll's contribution using a compression plate. In 13 out of 15 cases, the grafts were incorporated in an average of 13 weeks.

Oliveira discussed the use of iliac bone grafts in bone defects in 120 cases of chronic osteomyelitis. The object of treatment was to eliminate dead space after removal of infected soft tissues and sclerosed bone. **Meyer** described the results of treatment of infected un-united fractures by debridement of the soft tissue and bone and open suction drainage followed by rigid stabilisation and bone grafting. The late results showed good function and bone union in 60 out of 64 cases. The importance of local treatment of the infection prior to stabilisation of the fracture and the use of cancellous grafts is emphasised. **Kelly** clarified the surgical management of chronic osteomyelitis by removal of dead bone, obliteration of dead space and soft tissue coverage of exposed bone. He advocated the use of external fixation devices to treat unstable infected non-union. Muscle flaps have been re-introduced to obtain closure of saucerised wounds. The precise steps of the Papineau technique for replacement of bone defects in cases of open and infected fractures and pseudarthroses are illustrated by **Burny**.

Chapman has provided a useful recent comprehensive chapter on the various types of autogenous bone grafts and the techniques for harvesting these grafts.

Electrical Stimulation

Brighton CT, Black J, Friedenberg ZB, Esterhai JL, Day LJ, Connolly JF **A multi-center study of the treatment of non-union with constant direct current** J Bone Joint Surg [Am] 1981;63-A:2–13

Brighton CT **Current concepts review. The treatment of non-unions with electricity** J Bone Joint Surg [Am] 1981;63-A:847–851

Bassett CAL, Mitchell SN, Gaston SR **Treatment of ununited tibial diaphyseal fractures with pulsing electromagnetic fields** J Bone Joint Surg [Am] 1981; 63-A:511–523

The use of electrical stimulation in the treatment of non-union is still controversial. In the first of two papers, **Brighton** presented the results of a constant direct current for twelve weeks in 178 non-unions; 84% achieved solid bony union. Failure was due to inadequate electricity, a synovial pseudarthrosis, infection or a large gap at the fracture site. In the second paper laboratory and clinical studies were presented and the results of three systems, invasive, semi-invasive and non-invasive, compared. All three gave the same overall success rate and required the same time for healing. **Bassett** summarised the principles and techniques which he has evolved for the electromagnetic treatment of non-union of the tibia.

Vascularised Grafts

Weiland AJ **Current concepts review. Vascularised free bone transplants** J Bone Joint Surg [Am] 1981;63-A:166–169

Pho RWH, Vajara R, Satku K **Free vascularised bone transplants in problematic non-unions of fractures** J Trauma 1983;23:341–349

Chacha PB, Ahmed M, Daruwalla JS **Vascular pedicle graft of the ipsilateral fibula for non-union of the tibia with a large defect – an experimental and clinical study** J Bone Joint Surg [Br] 1981;63-B:244–253

Weiland has reviewed the traditional methods of bone grafting and advocated free vascularised bone grafts in carefully selected patients. Massive autogenous bone grafting with intact vascular pedicles decreased the time for bone union. Although only presenting three cases, **Pho** described his operative technique in detail. A new armamentarium has been introduced to solve a major reconstruction problem. The use of vascularised fibula grafts in eleven patients with a large tibial defect and sepsis is described by **Chacha**. The salvaged limbs were stiff and ugly, but the patients were free from pain, oedema, or persistent infection. These grafts provide a strong internal "live" splint and introduce a large vascular bed to the non-union site.

Open Fractures

Gustilo RB, Anderson JT **Prevention of infection in the treatment of 1025 open fractures of long bones – retrospective and prospective analysis** J Bone Joint Surg [Am] 1976;58-A:453–458

Gustilo RB, Gruninger RP, Davis T **Classification of Type III (severe) open fractures relative to treatment and results** Orthopaedics 1987;10:1781–1788

Chapman MW, Mahoney M **The role of early internal fixation in the management of open fractures** Clin Orthop 1979;138:120–131

Rittmann WW, Schibli M, Matter M, Allgower M **Open fractures: long-term results in 200 consecutive cases** Clin Orthop 1979;138:132–140

Schatzker J, Tile M **Open fractures**. In: The rationale of operative fracture care Berlin, etc: Springer-Verlag 1987:23–27

In 1976 **Gustilo** classified open fractures into three categories and this work has become the standard reference on this subject. The results of a prospective study of 352 open fractures with guide lines for treatment were presented. The infection rate was 2.5%. Cephalosporin was currently the prophylactic antibiotic of choice. In the type III fractures the infection rates were 44% in the retrospective study and 9% in the prospective study. Primary closure was indicated for type I and II open fractures.

In 1987 **Gustilo** divided type III fractures into three groups depending on the degree of soft tissue damage. The increasing rates of sepsis, non-union and amputation were described in the three sub-groups. A detailed summary presents principles in the treatment of open fractures with increasing emphasis on the use of early bone grafting.

Chapman carefully marshalled arguments in the controversy over the use of internal fixation in open fractures. Fixation is particularly indicated in multiple injuries, type III open fractures, massively traumatised limbs, vascular injuries, intra-articular fractures and some fractures in the elderly. The long-term results of treatment of two hundred consecutive patients is presented by **Rittmann**. Fractures were managed by AO principles and all, except one, united. **Schatzker** summarised modern management with a description of operative treatment, choice of fixation and implant selection. External fixation is indicated for grade III open wounds with severe comminution or bone loss in either the metaphysis or diaphysis.

External Fixation of Fractures

General Review

Behrens F **External fixation** Curr Orthop 1988;2:9–13

Biomechanics

Mooney V, Claudi B **How stable should external fixation be?** In: Uhthoff HK, ed. Current concepts of external fixation of fractures Berlin, etc: Springer-Verlag 1982:21–27

Methods

Section 4: External Fixation (Burny F and others) In: Ackroyd CE, O'Connor BT, Debruyn PF, ed. The severely injured limb Edinburgh, etc: Churchill Livingstone 1983:81–165

Campbell D, Kempson GF **Which external fixation device?** Injury 1980;12: 291–296

Complications

Green SA **Complications of external fixation** In: Uhthoff HK, ed. Current concepts of external fixation of fractures Berlin, etc: Springer-Verlag 1982:43–52

Treatment of Non-Union

Green SA **Septic non-union** In: Uhthoff HK, ed. Current concepts of external fixation of fractures Berlin, etc: Springer-Verlag 1982:221–233

Results

De Bastiani G, Aldgheri R, Renzibrivio L **The treatment of fractures with a dynamic axial fixator** J Bone Joint Surg [Br] 1984;66-B:538–545

Behrens has provided a short general review of this rapidly developing subject. **Mooney** discussed the biomechanics and pointed out that the history of development of external fixation has revolved around the question of the type of stability desired. Complete stability or stress shielding is an adverse condition for functional healing of fractures. The principles and biomechanics of external fixation are further discussed by **Burny** in the first part of the section on **External Fixation**. The remainder of this symposium consists of chapters on six of the more commonly used external fixators including the AO system, the Day frame and the Hoffman system. Seven external fixation frames which are used for the treatment of fractures have been evaluated by **Campbell** and the advantages and disadvantages of each, particularly in relation to versatility, stiffness and quality are described.

Complications of external fixation are considered by **Green**, particularly pin track infections, chronic pinhole osteomyelitis, failure to obtain union, neurovascular injury and persistent wound infection.

Green, in a further paper, considered the use of external skeletal fixation in septic non-union of long bones. The fixator allowed limb lengths to be maintained after resection of cortical bone. Access was provided for dressings and healing was promoted.

De Bastiani related experience with the treatment of a series of 338 fractures of major long bones and the pelvis. A high rate of union was obtained and there was a low incidence of pin track infections.

Pathological Fractures

General Principles

Wilson JN **Pathological fractures** In: Watson-Jones' fractures and joint injuries. Vol 2, 6th edn Edinburgh, etc: Churchill Livingstone 1982:1207–1280

11

Springfield DS, Brower TD **Pathologic fractures** In: Rockwood CA, Green DP ed. Fractures in adults Vol 1, 2nd edn Philadelphia, etc: JB Lippincott 1984:295–312

Smith R **Biochemical disorders of the skeleton** London: Butterworth 1979: (Osteoporosis) 71–94, (osteomalacia) 95–132, (Paget's disease of bone) 133–159, (osteogenesis imperfecta) 180–202

The chapter by **Wilson** has been chosen since it provides a general account of the wide variety of local and general disorders in which pathological fractures may occur. General principles of management are presented and the occurrence of pathological fractures in development and nutritional deficiencies, generalised bone diseases and primary benign and malignant tumours illustrated. **Springfield** is included since general evaluation of the patient is stressed and the chapter reflects increased interest in pathological fractures due to malignant disease. Sources of information on generalised bone diseases are often voluminous and scattered; we have repeatedly returned to the small book by **Smith** since it contains concise and easily read chapters on some of the common general conditions of bone such as osteoporosis, osteomalacia and osteogenesis imperfecta.

Malignant Disease

Galasko CSB **Local complications of skeletal metastases** In: Skeletal metastases London, etc: Butterworth 1986:128–155

Harrington KD, Sim FH, Enis JE, Johnston JO, Dick HM, Gristina AG **Methylmethacrylate as an adjunct to internal fixation of pathological fractures – experience with 375 patients** J Bone Joint Surg [Am] 1976; 58-A:1047–1055

Upper Limb Metastases

Sim FH, Pritchard DJ **Metastatic disease in the upper extremity** Clin Orthop 1982;169:83–94

Lower Limb Metastases

Harrington K **New trends in the management of lower extremity metastases** Clin Orthop 1982;169:53–61

Lane JM, Sculco TP, Zolan S **Treatment of pathological fractures of the hip by endoprosthetic replacement** J Bone Joint Surg [Am] 1980;62-A:954–959

Habermann ET, Sach R, Stern RE, Hirsh DM & Anderson WJ **The pathology and treatment of metastatic disease of the femur** Clin Orthop 1982;169:70–82

Zickel RE, Mouradian WH **Intramedullary fixation of pathological fractures and lesions of the sub-trochanteric region of the femur** J Bone Joint Surg [Am] 1976;58-A:1061–1066

Spinal Metastases

Harrington KD **Current concepts review. Metastatic disease of the spine** J Bone Joint Surg [Am] 1986;68-A:1110–1115

Fidler MW **Pathological fractures of the cervical spine – palliative surgical treatment** J Bone Joint Surg [Br] 1985;67-B:352–357

Galasko stressed the general principles of advances in management of pathological fractures. Treatment includes three aspects: the orthopaedic management, the use of localised irradiation and the treatment of the causative tumour. The development of an impending fracture, pathological fracture or spinal instability is not necessarily a terminal event. The aim of treatment is to alleviate pain and restore mobility and, with the exception of pathological trans-cervical femoral fractures, this is best achieved by internal stabilisation. The type of stabilisation depends on the site of the lesion. **Harrington** described the management of 375 pathological or impending fractures. Local tumour resection and internal fixation supplemented by intramedullary methylmethacrylate proved highly successful. Eighty-five per cent of patients had good relief of pain. Internal fixation was contra-indicated where the life expectancy was less than three months.

The various types of fixation possible for different fractures in the upper limb are discussed by **Sim**.

Metastases involving the pelvis and lower extremities are common. **Harrington** outlined trends in treatment for intertrochanteric and sub-trochanteric fractures and also fractures involving the acetabulum. Specialist fixation devices may be necessary. The management of 167 consecutive pathological or impending fractures of the hip treated by endoprosthetic replacement is discussed by **Lane**. There was a dramatic relief of pain in all patients. Either a long stem femoral endoprosthesis or a total prosthetic hip was used. Cementing the prosthesis allowed stabilisation of the entire femur as well as resection of diseased bone. Specific problems concerning the pathology and treatment of disease in the shaft of the femur are discussed by **Habermann**. The use of the **Zickel** nail without cement in 46 patients with 35 fractures and 11 impending fractures is described by the originator of this method of treatment. The device allows early weight bearing, lives may be prolonged and the paper illustrates the general trend towards a more aggressive approach in the management of these fractures with the support of improved radiotherapy or chemotherapy.

Harrington has reviewed the problems of management of metastatic disease in the spine. Patients who have evidence of spinal metastases without vertebral collapse and without neurological impairment should have chemotherapy or hormonal treatment. He recommended operative decompression, usually anteriorly, and stabilisation for certain patients who have spinal metastases and intractable pain. **Fidler** has discussed the management of these problems in the cervical spine. Eleven patients had operations for severe pain due to a pathological fracture which, in eight of the cases, was unstable. Conservative treatment had either failed or was unsuitable.

Myelomatosis

Griffiths DL **Orthopaedic aspects of myelomatosis** J Bone Joint Surg [Br] 1966; 48-B:703–728

Goodman MA **Plasma cell tumours** Clin Orthop 1986;204:86–92

Griffiths studied 243 patients with myelomatosis and provided a comprehensive analysis of the local and general manifestations of the disease, presenting symptoms, the appearance of pathological fractures, the changes in the blood and prognosis. A modern appraisal of treatment and prognosis is summarised by **Goodman**. Primary treatment is by chemotherapy. A small number of patients present with pathological fractures that require stabilisation, sometimes with adjunctive methylmethacrylate.

Paget's Disease

Barry HC **Fractures**. In: Paget's disease of bone Edinburgh, etc: E & S Livingstone 1969:105–135

Dove J **Complete fractures of the femur in Paget's disease of bone** J Bone Joint Surg [Br] 1980;62-B:12–17

Smith R **Paget's disease of bone** In: Biochemical disorders of the skeleton London, etc: Butterworth 1979:133–159

The monograph by **Barry** presented a description of Paget's original cases and a prac-tical chapter describing the characteristics and results of treatment of fractures in this condition. A retrospective study of 182 fractures of the femur in Paget's disease is describ-ed by **Dove**. The incidence of non-union was 40%, the main problems being posed by the sub-trochanteric fractures and those of the upper shaft of the femur. **Smith** has described a general analysis of Paget's disease of bone including the pathology and cli-nical aspects, radiology and treatment. Fractures in association with this condition receive small mention but the chapter is included particularly for its observations on treatment, the possible use of calcitonin and diphosphonates. In 1877 Paget considered the disease to be an inflammation of the bones and suggested that "for brief reference and for the present, it may be called after its most striking character, osteitis deformans. A better name may be given when more is known of it". Despite the hopes expressed by Paget, over 100 years ago, the cause of this disease is still not known.

Osteoporosis and Fractures

Smith R **Osteoporosis**. In: Biochemical disorders of the skeleton London, etc: Butterworth 1979:71–94

Lane JM, Vigorita VJ **Current concepts review osteoporosis** J Bone Joint Surg [Am] 1983;65-A:274–278

Riggs BL, Melton LJ **Evidence for two distinct syndromes of involutional osteoporosis** AJM 1983;75:144–149

Smith R **Osteoporosis – cause and management** Br Med J 1987;294:329–333

Chalmers J, Ho KC **Geographical variations in senile osteoporosis – the association with physical activity** J Bone Joint Surg [Br] 1970;52-B:667–675

Jenson GF, Christiansen C, Boesen J, Hegedus V, Transbol I **Epidemiology of post-menopausal spinal and long bone fractures – a unifying approach to post-menopausal osteoporosis** Clin Orthop 1982;166:75–81

Aitken M **Osteoporosis in clinical practice** Bristol: J Wright 1984: (osteoporosis: related fractures) 70–87, (investigation of the osteoporotic patient) 87–93, (management of osteoporosis) 94–110

The authors have been particularly conscious of their task in this section. There are a huge number of papers on osteoporosis which are largely of interest to the physician, epidemiologist or pathologist. We have chosen a small number providing general reviews for the orthopaedic surgeon.

The causes of osteoporosis are classified by **Smith**, measurement of bone mass discussed and the clinical aspects summarised. The treatment, including both prevention and therapy of established osteoporosis, is outlined. Up-to-date knowledge on the pathophysiology of loss of bone mass is discussed by **Lane**. The difficulties of treatment which are described as still not satisfactory are outlined.

Two types of osteoporosis have been described by **Riggs**; it occurs in post-menopausal women from ages about 51 to 65 and this group sustain fractures such as those at the wrist and the vertebrae; the other type occurs in patients older than 75 years and these patients sustain fractures of the neck of the femur. The female to male ratio of incidence is six to one in the younger group but only two to one in the older group. The first group is considered to be due to loss of trabecular bone whilst the second is due to loss of both trabecular and cortical bone.

Smith has produced a recent update (1987) on the causes of osteoporosis described quite simply as old age, senility and the menopause. The current debate on possible prevention and management is presented. Oestrogens do prevent bone loss and reduce fracture rate in post-menopausal women but the disproportionate increase in the rate of femoral neck fractures is still not explained.

Chalmers noted that the incidence of senile osteoporosis is found to vary greatly in

15

different racial groups. The possibility that the occurrence of senile osteoporosis is related to reduced physical activity is discussed.

A detailed study of fractures of the spine with osteoporosis is described by **Jensen**. There are two types of fracture – the wedge and the crush. Some workers have considered that the crush fracture is the only reliable radiological evidence of spinal osteoporosis.

There are a number of books on osteoporosis. We have chosen that by **Aitken** since it is relatively small and has several relevant useful chapters for the orthopaedic surgeon; there is one specifically on related fractures, another on the investigations of the osteoporotic patient and finally one on the management of osteoporosis.

Osteomalacia and Fractures

Chalmers J, Conacher WDH, Gardner DL, Scott PJ **Osteomalacia – a common disease in elderly women** J Bone Joint Surg [Br] 1967;49-B:403–423

Smith R **Osteomalacia.** In: Biochemical disorders of the skeleton London, etc: Butterworth 1979:95–132

Mankin HJ **Review article. Rickets, osteomalacia, and renal osteodystrophy.** Part 1. J Bone Joint Surg [Am] 1974;56-A:101–128

Chalmers studied in detail 37 cases. Skeletal pain is noted to be the most constant symptom. Muscle weakness is a marked feature of the severe cases. Complete fractures are less characteristic of osteomalacia than they are of osteoporosis. Looser's zones are described. The pathology, aetiology and treatment are discussed. **Smith** has summarised recent advances. In rickets and osteomalacia the cardinal abnormality is defective mineralisation of bone and the main cause a lack of Vitamin D or a disturbance of its metabolism. Although osteomalacia is stated to be uncommon, it is disabling and responds well to treatment. Awareness of the diagnosis is therefore important. A review article on rickets, osteomalacia and renal osteodystrophy was published by **Mankin** in 1974. This is a classic reference article but it does specifically discuss the common fractures in this condition (pp. 118–119) and the milkman's syndrome, a ribbon-like pseudo-fracture of the long and flat bones without displacement or callus formation.

Stress Fractures

Devas MB **Stress fractures of the femoral neck** J Bone Joint Surg [Br] 1965; 47-B:728–738

Devas MB **Stress fractures** Edinburgh, etc: Churchill Livingstone 1975

Prather JL, Nusynowitz ML, Snowdy HA, Hughes AD, McCartney WH, Bagg RJ **Scintigraphic findings in stress fractures** J Bone Joint Surg [Am] 1977; 59-A:869–874

Kaltas D-S **Stress fractures of the femoral neck in young adults – a report of seven cases** J Bone Joint Surg [Br] 1981:63-B:33–37

Milgrom C, Giladi M, Stein M, Kashtan H, Margulies JY, Chisin R, Steinberg R, Aharonson Z **Stress fractures in military recruits – a prospective study showing an unusually high incidence** J Bone Joint Surg [Br] 1985;67-B:732–735

Devas has made a special study of stress fractures and their problems. Twenty-five patients were described with stress fractures of the femoral neck in one of his early papers in 1965. Distinction was made between compression and transverse fractures and it was emphasised that the transverse stress fracture may become displaced and therefore must be recognised. In 1975 **Devas** published a comprehensive monograph with chapters on stress fractures of particularly the fibula, tibia, femur and pelvis. Judging by the literature, the subject does not appear to be a particularly topical one at the present time. **Prather** studied scintigraphic findings in stress fractures and noted that in some patients the radiographs were normal whilst the scintigram was positive. **Kaltas** has drawn attention to stress fractures of the femoral neck in seven young adults. They were all young recruits undergoing military training. Finally, in a prospective study of 295 male Israeli military recruits, **Milgrom** found a 31% incidence of stress fractures. Eighty per cent of these were in the tibia or femoral shaft while only 8% occurred in the tarsus and metatarsus.

Pathological Fractures of the Hand

Noble J, Potts H **Pathological fractures of the hand** In: Barton NJ, ed. Fractures of the hand and wrist. Edinburgh, etc: Churchill Livingstone 1988:136–144

A pathological fracture in the hand is rare and is most likely to be secondary to an enchondroma. **Noble** has reviewed possible causes and management.

Vascular Injuries

Major Arterial

Ashton F, Slaney G **Arterial injuries in civilian surgical practice** Injury 1970;1:303–313

17

Connolly J **Management of fractures associated with arterial injuries** Surgery 1971;120:331

Eadie DGA **Editorial: Post-traumatic ischaemia** J Bone Joint Surg [Br] 1979; 61-B:265–266

Barros D'Sa AAB **A decade of missile-induced vascular trauma** Ann R Coll Surg Engl 1982;64:37–44

Birnstingl M **Vascular injuries** In: Wilson JN, ed. Watson-Jones' fractures and joint injuries. 6th edn Vol. 1 Edinburgh, etc: Churchill Livingstone 1982:211–241

Simms MH **Management of vascular injuries** In: Alpar EK, Owen R, ed. Paediatric trauma: Tunbridge Wells: Castle House Publications 1988:107–123

Ashton reviewed 91 cases of arterial injury treated in Birmingham, England. Early diagnosis or exploration is essential and the time between injury and repair decisive. A diagnosis is nearly always possible on clinical signs and it should be assumed that an injury is present until proven absent. Arterial spasm should only be diagnosed after negative exploration. **Connolly** discussed problems of management of combined fracture and arterial injuries. The method of fracture management found most effective in Vietnam under field conditions was external immobilisation with casts or splints. Under more ideal conditions in civilian life, urgent internal fixation of the fracture provides a more satisfactory stabilisation and safeguards the vascular repair. Internal fixation increased the time for surgery and speed was essential. **Eadie** stressed the importance of early diagnosis of occlusion of major peripheral artery for the fate of the limb. Experience in Belfast is narrated by **Barros D'Sa** over a ten-year period. The importance of meticulous repair, timely fasciotomy and early re-intervention is stressed and the amputation rate only 5%. **Birnstingl** has provided a general reference chapter with illustrations of surgical technique and the management of vascular injuries in children is discussed by **Simms.**

Compartment Syndromes

Mubarak SJ, Owen CA, Hargens AR, Garetto LP, Akeson WH **Acute compartment syndromes: diagnosis and treatment with the aid of the wick catheter** J Bone Joint Surg [Am] 1978;60-A:1091–1095

Mubarak SJ, Owen CA **Double-incision fasciotomy of the leg for decompression of compartment syndromes** J Bone Joint Surg [Am] 1977;59-A:184–187

Matsen FA, Winquist RA, Krugmire RB **Diagnosis and management of compartmental syndromes** J Bone Joint Surg [Am] 1980;62-A:286–291

Rorabeck CH The treatment of compartment syndromes of the leg J Bone Joint Surg [Br] 1984;66-B:93–97

Allan MJ, Stirling AJ, Crawshaw CV, Barnes MR Intra-compartmental pressure monitoring of leg injuries: an aid to management J Bone Joint Surg [Br] 1985;67-B:53–57

During the last 10 or 15 years there has been a growing appreciation of the importance of a compartment syndrome. **Mubarak** in 1978 stated "the sequelae of a compartment syndrome may be devastating – Volkmann's contracture, neural deficit, and even gangrene". He studied pressures using a Wick catheter technique in 65 compartments of 27 patients suspected of having an acute compartment syndrome. A pressure of 30mm Hg or more was an indication for decompressive fasciotomy. A catheter may be useful where the patient is uncooperative or unresponsive perhaps due to other injuries. **Mubarak**, in another paper, recommended a double-incision technique for fasciotomy of the leg for compartment syndromes. He considered this technique to be quicker and safer and therefore the treatment of choice. The procedure has advantages over localised removal of the fibula.

Matsen described a practical approach to the patient at risk and an infusion technique for measuring tissue pressure. He considered that patients with a pressure less than 45mm Hg did not require fasciotomy. If the pressure was 55mm Hg or more, surgery was required. The frequency and severity of complications were inversely related to the promptness of fasciotomy. **Rorabeck** described experience with 18 patients with an acute compartment syndrome in the leg. The most common symptom was pain over the affected compartment and the most common sign was pain on stretching the damaged muscles. **Allan** noted that acute compartment syndromes often develop insidiously and are recognised too late to prevent permanent disability. He studied continuous pressure monitoring as an aid to management in 28 patients and discussed the possible value of this technique.

Volkmann's Contracture

Seddon HJ Volkmann's contracture: treatment by excision of the infarct J Bone Joint Surg [Br] 1956;38-B:152–174

Seddon HJ Volkmann's ischaemia in the lower limb J Bone Joint Surg [Br] 1966;48-B:627–636

Holden CEA The pathology and prevention of Volkmann's ischaemic contracture J Bone Joint Surg [Br] 1979;61-B:296–300

Mubarak SJ, Carroll NC Volkmann's contracture in children: aetiology and prevention J Bone Joint Surg [Br] 1979;61-B:285–293

In 1956 **Seddon** described the presentation of 16 cases of Volkmann's contracture affecting the forearm flexors. He believed that the pathology was a massive muscular infarct and that in the established case this required treatment by excision. Possible aetiology was mentioned but prevention was not discussed. In a later article, also by **Seddon,** problems presented in the lower limb were outlined including the resulting deformity. The effects of ischaemia of nerves were described in both papers. These two classical papers provide basic information concerning this condition affecting the arm and the leg.

Holden has summarised the recent change in emphasis concerning the pathology and prevention of Volkmann's ischaemic contracture. Following direct injury to a limb, swelling occurs and ischaemia may result. If this develops in an unyielding osteofascial compartment, then contracture may result if not relieved by a timely fasciotomy. Experimental evidence for these observations is produced and the early diagnosis of compartment ischaemia outlined. It is stressed that pain may be an overriding symptom and that the diagnosis of this type of ischaemia can usually be made on clinical examination alone. In an adjacent article **Mubarak** described experience with 55 children, admitted over a period of twenty years to the Sick Children's Hospital in Toronto, with Volkmann's contracture in 58 limbs. Most of the children reviewed had not had early appropriate treatment. The frequency of this contracture had not declined in spite of many published reports on the compartment syndrome. It was concluded that there is still no room for complacency in the management of vascular injuries of the limbs which may complicate fractures.

Peripheral Nerve Injuries

General Review

Birch R **Lesions of peripheral nerves: the present position. In: Symposium on peripheral nerve injuries** J Bone Joint Surg [Br] 1986;68-B:2–8

Wynn Parry CB **Sensation. In: Symposium on peripheral nerve injuries** J Bone Joint Surg [Br] 1986;68-B:15–19

Bonney G **Iatrogenic injuries of nerves. In: Symposium on peripheral nerve injuries** J Bone Joint Surg [Br] 1986;68-B:9–13

Millesi H **Microsurgery of peripheral nerves.** In: McKibbin B ed. Recent advances in orthopaedics. Vol 4 Edinburgh, etc: Churchill Livingstone 1983:1–22

Seddon Sir HJ **Surgical disorders of the peripheral nerves.** 2nd edn Edinburgh, etc: Churchill Livingstone, 1975

Assessment

Moberg E **Objective methods for determining the functional value of sensibility in the hand** J Bone Joint Surg [Br] 1958;40-B:454–476

Omer GE **Injuries to nerves of the upper extremity** J Bone Joint Surg [Am] 1974;56-A:1615–1624

Birch's paper on the present position of lesions of peripheral nerves begins a recent symposium on this subject (1986). A concise review is presented of primary and delayed repair and of nerve grafting. Some special problems, including damage to the median nerve and methods of recording return of function, are discussed. **Wynn Parry** stressed that sensation must be assessed functionally and only then can the results of different techniques of nerve suture and grafts be truly compared. Excellent function may be regained even though two point discrimination remains grossly abnormal. The fascinating paper by **Bonney** on iatrogenic injuries of nerves will act as a reminder to all surgeons, no matter how experienced, of the increasing problems of legal aspects of accidental nerve damage. The chapter by **Millesi** summarised the development of microsurgical techniques and indicated continuing change in the philosophy of nerve repair. Surgery has become more delicate and results have been improved. **Seddon**'s classical textbook has been included as a standard reference. There are useful sections on electrical phenomena and methods of examination, lesions of the sciatic nerve and nerve injuries causing pain.

    Moberg observed clinically that the tactile gnosis varies directly with the sudomotor function of the hand. He described a practical procedure for determining the functional value of the cutaneous sensibility in the hand. **Omer** studied 917 nerve injuries over a five-year period. Spontaneous recovery occurred in 70% of gunshot wounds and 85% of fracture dislocations. Nerve suture was most successful in young patients less than 20-years of age.

Surgery

Jabaley M **Technical aspects of peripheral nerve repair** J Hand Surg 1984; 9-B:14–19

Kline DG **Timing for exploration of nerve lesions and evaluation of the neuroma – in continuity** Clin Orthop 1982;163:42–50

Braun RM **Epineurial nerve suture** Clin Orthop 1982;163:50–56

Urbaniak JR **Fascicular nerve suture** Clin Orthop 1982;163:57–64

Cabaud HE, Rodkey WG, McCarroll HR, Mutz SB, Niebauer JJ **Epineurial and perineurial fascicular nerve repairs: a critical comparison** J Hand Surg 1976;1:131–137

Millesi H, Meissl G, Berger A **The interfascicular nerve grafting of the median and ulnar nerves** J Bone Joint Surg [Am] 1972;54-A:727–750

Marsh D, Barton NJ **Does the use of the operating microscope improve the results of peripheral nerve suture?** J Bone Joint Surg [Br] 1987;69-B:625–630

Operative Technique

Birch R **The primary and secondary repair of divided peripheral nerves** In: Birch R, Brooks D, ed. The hand 4th edn, (Rob and Smith's Operative Surgery) London: Butterworth 1984:168–177

Fisher TR **Intrafascicular nerve grafting** In: Birch R, Brooks D, ed. The hand 4th edn, (Rob and Smith's Operative Surgery) London: Butterworth 1984:178–183

Reconstruction

Omer GE **Reconstructive procedures for extremities with peripheral nerve defects** Clin Orthop 1982;163:80–91

Payan J **Electromyographer's view of the ulnar nerve In: Symposium on peripheral nerve injuries** J Bone Joint Surg [Br] 1986;68-B:13–15

The anatomy of degeneration and regeneration and the principles of nerve repair were discussed by **Jabaley**. The difficult subject of the surgical evaluation of lesions in continuity and the use of a nerve stimulator is discussed by **Kline**. **Braun**'s paper on epineurial nerve suture is followed by **Urbaniak**'s on the fascicular nerve suture. Both are concise and practical and favour the epineurial repair for most nerve lesions. **Cabaud** showed in experimental acute nerve lacerations in the cat that epineurial neurorrhaphy is as satisfactory as intrafascicular perineurial neurorrhaphy. **Millesi** discussed the operative technique of nerve grafting and reviewed the results of 202 nerve grafts for median and ulnar nerve division. He concluded that nerve grafting without tension gave better results than end-to-end suture under tension and that microscopic repair is required. **Marsh** addressed the subject of the value of the operating microscope in possibly improving results of peripheral nerve suture. In a relatively small number of cases it was concluded that, in the hands of one particular surgeon, the use of the operating microscope gave no better results than careful epineurial suture performed without it.

Practical details of exposure, primary and secondary repair of divided peripheral nerves and intrafascicular nerve grafts are provided by **Birch** and **Fisher**.

Omer described the evaluation of patients requiring reconstructive procedures after peripheral nerve defects. Various tendon transfers which are available for each nerve injury are debated and it is stressed that gnosis is very important as "a sensory feed back for precise function". The paper on electromyography by **Payan** is concerned with the ulnar nerve but it has been included since it discussed the electromyographer's contribution to the management of nerve injuries.

Sudeck's Atrophy

The Classic

Plewes LW **Sudeck's atrophy in the hand** J Bone Joint Surg [Br] 1956; 38-B:195–203

Clinical Studies

Poplawski ZJ, Wiley AM, Murray JF **Post-traumatic dystrophy of the extremities: a clinical review and trial of treatment** J Bone Joint Surg [Am] 1983;65-A:642–655

Katz MM, Hungerford DS **Reflex sympathetic dystrophy affecting the knee** J Bone Joint Surg [Br] 1987;69-B:797–803

Schutzer SF, Gossling HR **Current concepts review: the treatment of reflex sympathetic dystrophy syndrome** J Bone Joint Surg [Am] 1984;66-A:625–629

This troublesome condition was first described by Sudeck in the German literature in 1900. The name "reflex sympathetic dystrophy syndrome" has become popular recently but this implies a certainty of aetiology which is not proven. **Plewes** described and illustrated the characteristic presentation and stressed that conservative treatment by heat, elevation and graded function is effective if initiated early within six weeks of the onset of symptoms.

Poplawski and **Katz** noted that the condition affects structures other than the hand; they stress that early diagnosis remains the key to successful management and the importance of breaking the vicious pain cycle that is characteristic of the syndrome. **Schutzer** discussed the various modalities of treatment including the use of steroids and provides a useful reference list for further reading.

Paediatric Trauma: General Aspects

Basic Anatomy and Fracture Healing

McKibbin B **The structure of the epiphysis** In: Owen R, Goodfellow J, Bullough P, ed. Orthopaedics and traumatology London: William Heinemann Medical Books 1980;169–175

Weber BG **Fracture healing in the growing bone and in the mature skeleton**. In: Weber BG, Brunner Ch, Freuler F, ed. The treatment of fractures in children and adolescents Berlin, etc: Springer-Verlag, 1980:20–57

The Growth Plate

Salter RB, Harris WR **Injuries involving the epiphyseal plate** J Bone Joint Surg [Am] 1963;45-A:587–622

Rang M **Injuries of the epiphysis, growth plate and perichondrial ring** In: Rang M, ed. Children's fractures, 2nd edn. Philadelphia: JB Lippincott, 1983:10–25

Langenskiold A **An operation for partial closure of an epiphyseal plate in children and its experimental basis** J Bone Joint Surg [Br] 1975;57-B:325–330

Ogden JA **Current concepts review: the evaluation and treatment of partial physeal arrest** J Bone Joint Surg [Am] 1987;69-A:1297–1302

A basic reference has been provided to the structure of the epiphysis including the growth plate by **McKibbin**. **Weber** compared the healing of shaft fractures in growing bone with mature bone and discussed functional adaptation following a fracture.

Considerable interest has recently been shown in disorders of the growth plate. The classical paper by **Salter** on the different types of injury is now a standard reference and gives a clear description of the types of injury, possible causes of altered growth and its nature. **Rang** has more recently amplified and illustrated the basic anatomy and discussed injuries at the growth plate. **Langenskiold** has spent a lifetime studying premature fusion and its possible surgical treatment. He has shown that excision of a bony bridge and replacement with fat can prevent recurrence of the bridge. **Ogden** has recently summarised these developments, discussing the various types of bridge formation, the technique of resection and the materials that may be used for interposition and the results of this surgery.

Growth Changes in Long Bones

Reynolds DA **Growth changes in fractured long bones – a study of 126 children** J Bone Joint Surg [Br] 1981;63-B:83–88

Remodelling

Rang M **Remodelling** In: Children's fractures. 2nd edn Philadelphia: JB Lippincott, 1983:31–32

Principles of Management

Alpar EK, Owen R **General considerations and principles of management** In: Paediatric trauma Tunbridge Wells: Castle House Publications, 1988:1–17

Spontaneous correction of shortening with growth after fractures of the long bones in children is now universally recognised. **Reynolds** studied this problem in 126 children over some years. Within three months of injury, the rate of growth was at its maximum and was 38% in excess of normal. The greatest rate of growth occurred after injuries which resulted in overlap of the fragments.

It is seldom easy to predict accurately what remodelling will accomplish in the older child. **Rang** provided some general principles indicating when remodelling will help in the restoration of normal anatomy. Remodelling is particularly valuable in children with at least two years of growth remaining, in fractures near the ends of long bones and to correct deformity in the plane of movement of a joint.

In a recent chapter, **Alpar** (1988) has summarised the principles of management of musculo-skeletal injuries in children. There is growing awareness of the need for open reduction of some fractures in children and these are listed.

Child Abuse

Akbarnia B, Torg JS, Kirkpatrick J, Sussman S **Manifestations of the battered-child syndrome** J Bone Joint Surg [Am] 1974;56-A:1159–1166

Editorial **Child abuse: the swing of the pendulum** Br Med J 1981;283:170

Galleno H, Oppenheim WL **The battered child syndrome revisited** Clin Orthop 1982;162:11–19

Roberton DM, Barbor P, Hull D **Unusual injury? Recent injury in normal children and children with suspected non-accidental injury** Br Med J 1982; 285:1399–1401

Hobbs CJ **Skull fracture and the diagnosis of abuse** Arch Dis Child 1984;59: 246–252

Since the term "battered child syndrome" was introduced by Kempe in 1962, there has been a growing awareness that many traumatic injuries suffered by children are not accidental in origin. **Akbarnia** showed that of 217 children admitted, one-third required orthopaedic treatment. This paper discussed the prevalence of the syndrome, the orthopaedic and non-orthopaedic manifestations, and the surgeon's responsibilities to the battered child and the child's family.

An **editorial** in the British Medical Journal in 1981 stressed that whilst missing a definite case may be tragic, so also was a false accusation and judging whether abuse has taken place may be one of the most difficult and agonising decisions a doctor has to make. The social aspects of the management of these difficult injuries is discussed and it is emphasised there may be a mortality rate of 10% and a recurrence rate of 60%.

Galleno in 1982 presented a study of 66 children and stressed the importance of the specific nature of the fracture (such as bilaterality or corner metaphyseal fractures) rather than the old addage of "three fractures in different stages of healing". Clues are tabled which may assist in making a proper diagnosis. **Roberton** compared the effects of recent injury in normal children and in children with suspected non-accidental injury. In those with non-accidental injury, 60% had injuries to the head and face and this increase in prevalence was seen in children of all ages. These children also had more frequent injuries in the lumbar region, particularly before the age of five years. There may be obligation to report the case to authorities outside of the treatment facility.

Hobbs has pointed out the importance of skull fractures in this condition. The characteristics of such fractures in abused children were multiple or complex configuration, depressed or wide fractures. There was sometimes involvement of more than one cranial bone.

Tetanus and Gas Gangrene

Tetanus

Edmondson RS **Tetanus** Br J Hosp Med 1980;23:596–602

Gas Gangrene

Altemeier WA, Fullen WD **Prevention and treatment of gas gangrene** JAMA 1971;217:806–813

Colwill MR, Maudsley RH **The management of gas gangrene with hyperbaric oxygen therapy** J Bone Joint Surg [Br] 1968;50-B:732–742

Tetanus is now a rare infection in the Western world. **Edmondson** presented a comprehensive study discussing the pathogenesis, prophylaxis, diagnosis and treatment. Important advances in treatment with anti-tetanus serum are described. He stressed the severity and how the treatment regime for each grade can vary. Even with intensive care in Western countries, the reported mortality may vary from nil to 60%.

Altemeier summarised the prevention and treatment of gas gangrene and included a section discussing the non-clostridial lesions that can simulate gas gangrene. Success of treatment is dependent on urgent diagnosis in view of the rapidity of the spread of infection. It was concluded that at present no treatment has replaced early extensive surgery in the treatment of gas gangrene. **Colwill** described the management of gas gangrene by hyperbaric oxygen. The mode of action and administration and risks are discussed. A series of 17 cases, with one death, is recorded from a hospital unit with a small chamber using two atmospheres in pure oxygen.

Brachial Plexus Injuries

General Review

Seddon Sir HJ **Surgical disorders of the peripheral nerves.** 2nd edn Edinburgh, etc: Churchill Livingstone 1975;174–198

Wynn Parry CB **Brachial plexus injuries** Br J Hosp Med 1984;32:130–139

Birch R **Traction lesions of the brachial plexus** Br J Hosp Med 1984;32:140–143

Investigation

Marshall RW, De Silva RDD **Computerised axial tomography in traction injuries of the brachial plexus** J Bone Joint Surg [Br] 1986;68-B:734–738

Surgery

Narakas A **Surgical treatment of traction injuries of the brachial plexus** Clin Orthop 1978;133:71–90

Sedel L **The results of surgical repair of brachial plexus injuries** J Bone Joint Surg [Br] 1982;64-B:54–66

Follow-Up

Ransford AO, Hughes SPF **Complete brachial plexus lesions: A 10-year follow-up 20 cases** J Bone Joint Surg [Br] 1977;59-B:417–420

Infraclavicular Injuries

Leffert RD, Seddon Sir HJ **Infraclavicular brachial plexus injuries** J Bone Joint Surg [Br] 1965;47-B:9–22

Rehabilitation

Wynn Parry CB **Rehabilitation of the hand.** 4th edn London: Butterworth 1981:134–146, 157–180, 348–354

Seddon has provided standard textbook knowledge with special reference to surgical anatomy and the types of injury suffered. The papers by **Wynn Parry** and **Birch** update the considerable advances made on this subject.

Myelography often underestimates the severity of the lesion and electrophysiology is a vital element in the assessment of patients in the operating theatre. More extensive operative explorations have given a more precise recognition of distal lesions. A benefit conferred by early exploration is the availability of a reasonably accurate prognosis.

Marshall's paper on CT scanning superseded the classic 1968 paper by Yeoman and compared CT scanning with conventional myelography and surgical exploration. Enhanced CTs correlated well with operative findings and improved diagnostic accuracy particularly at the fifth and sixth root levels.

In 1978 **Narakas** described experience with the results of operative treatment in 105 patients. In about 10% no reconstruction was possible. There was a striking difference in results of supraclavicular and distal infraclavicular lesions. **Sedel**'s paper presented an analysis of the results of surgery in 63 patients, approximately half with complete and half with partial lesions, and provided a clear protocol for examination and repair; results are discussed with a three-year follow-up of direct suture, nerve grafting and later neurolysis.

Ransford's paper on complete brachial plexus lesions provided a 9 $1/2$-year follow-up of 20 patients. Changing attitudes to treatment are clearly described. Amputation does not relieve the distressing symptom of severe pain, should not be considered until a year after injury and only for a clearly defined reason.

The paper on infraclavicular lesions by **Leffert** described those occurring as a direct result of skeletal injury in the region of the shoulder joint, discussed the good prognosis and advocated conservative management.

Wynn Parry has contributed particularly on the management of severe and characteristic chronic pain from which these patients may suffer. The most valuable treatment for pain is transcutaneous nerve stimulation. The indications for amputation and programme for long-term rehabilitation are discussed. Functional splinting improves these patients' function at both work and hobbies.

The authors are conscious that a number of well known classics have not been included in this presentation, e.g. Bonney (1959) and Yeoman and Seddon (1961); they have been omitted because of the complete change now occurring in the attitude to management of these difficult and often distressing problems.

Fractures of the Clavicle

The Classics

Rowe CR **An atlas of anatomy and treatment of mid-clavicular fractures** Clin Orthop 1968;58:29–42

Neer CS **Non-union of the clavicle** JAMA 1960;172:1006–1011

Surgical Treatment

Neer CS **Fractures of distal third of the clavicle** Clin Orthop 1968;58:43–50

Zenni EJ, Krieg JK, Rosen MJ **Open reduction and internal fixation of clavicular fractures** J Bone Joint Surg [Am] 1981;63-A:147–151

29

Rowe studied 690 fractures of the clavicle, stressed the very low incidence of non-union when treated conservatively but nevertheless included rare indications for open reduction. **Neer** described a study of 18 collected cases of non-union. Of 14 patients with fractures of the middle third, ten had been treated initially by operation.

In 1968, **Neer** described the pathological anatomy of the lateral third fracture, the higher incidence of non-union at this site and the difficulties of management. **Zenni** has recently provided a practical article clarifying the rare indications for operative treatment and illustrating his technique.

Injuries of the Sternoclavicular Joint

Salvatore JE **Sternoclavicular joint dislocation** Clin Orthop 1968;58:51–55

We have traced one paper discussing anterior and posterior dislocation at the sternoclavicular joint and include this for rapid reference. Fourteen sternoclavicular dislocations are presented for study.

Injuries of the Acromioclavicular Joint

Classification

Rockwood CA, Green DP **Fractures in adults**. 2nd edn, Vol.1 Philadelphia: JB Lippincott 1984:860–910

Treatment

Copeland S, Kessel L **Disruption of the acromioclavicular joint: surgical anatomy and biological reconstruction** Injury 1979;11:208–214

Larson E, Bjerg-Nielson A, Christensen P **Conservative or surgical treatment of acromioclavicular dislocation** J Bone Joint Surg [Am] 1986;68-A:552–555

Dias JJ, Steingold RF, Richardson RA, Tesfayohannes B, Gregg PJ **The conservative treatment of acromioclavicular dislocation – review after five years** J Bone Joint Surg [Br] 1987;69-B:719–722

The pathological anatomy and classification are described and illustrated in the textbook by **Rockwood** and also by **Copeland**. There is little discussion on the best method of treating those with minor displacement (types I and II injuries), but the best treatment for type III injuries has been debated for years and the saga looks likely to continue. **Larson** described the results of a prospective controlled randomised study comparing conservative and surgical treatment. The papers mentioned describe two types of fixation and repair, either across the acromio-clavicular joint or with a screw into the coracoid. Fixation into the coracoid is now probably the more popular of the two methods and it is interesting to note that this was originally described by Bosworth as a technique under local anaesthesia! A long-term follow-up of type III injuries treated conservatively has been published by **Dias** and he found good results in 43 out of 44 patients. The general impression which is supported by these papers is that there is probably little to be gained by acute surgical repair except, rarely, in the athlete or heavy manual worker.

Dislocations of the Shoulder Joint

The Classic

Rowe CR **Prognosis in dislocations of the shoulder** J Bone Joint Surg [Am] 1956;38-A:957–977

Pre-Operative Assessment

Gerber C, Ganz R **Clinical assessment of instability of the shoulder. With special reference to anterior and posterior drawer tests** J Bone Joint Surg [Br] 1984;66-B:551–556

Recurrent Anterior Dislocation

Osmond-Clarke H **Habitual dislocation of the shoulder. The Putti-Platt operation** J Bone Joint Surg [Br] 1948;30-B:19–25

Adams JC **Recurrent dislocation of the shoulder** J Bone Joint Surg [Br] 1948; 30-B:26–38

Rowe CR, Patel D, Southmayd WW **The Bankart procedure. A long-term end-result study** J Bone Joint Surg [Am] 1978;60-A:1–16

Hovelius L, Korner L, Lundberg B, Akermark C, Herberts P, Wredmark T, Berg E **The coracoid transfer for recurrent dislocation of the shoulder. Technical aspects of the Bristow-Latarjet procedure** J Bone Joint Surg [Am] 1983; 65-A:926–934

Karadimas J, Rentis G, Varouchas G **Repair of recurrent anterior dislocation of the shoulder using transfer of the subscapularis tendon** J Bone Joint Surg [Am] 1980;62-A:1147–1149

Leslie JT, Ryan TJ **The anterior axillary incision to approach the shoulder joint** J Bone Joint Surg [Am] 1962;44-A:1193–1196

The Unreduced Dislocation

Rowe CR, Zarins B **Chronic unreduced dislocations of the shoulder** J Bone Joint Surg [Am] 1982;64-A:494–505

Posterior Dislocation

Nobel W **Posterior traumatic dislocation of the shoulder** J Bone Joint Surg [Am] 1962;44-A:523–538

McLaughlin HL **Posterior dislocation of the shoulder** J Bone Joint Surg [Am] 1952;34-A:584–590

Nerve Injury

Leffert RD, Seddon Sir HJ **Infraclavicular brachial plexus injuries** J Bone Joint Surg [Br] 1965;47-B:9–22

In 1956 **Rowe** published a study of 488 patients suffering from dislocation of the shoulder and this analysed in detail basic information such as the types and incidence of dislocation, associated humeral head defects, and complications. It is perhaps noteworthy that there was a specialised clinic in Boston in 1956 for problems of the shoulder and this reflects the continued concentrated interest shown on these problems in the USA.

Gerber's paper drew attention to the difficulty sometimes experienced in assessment of anterior and posterior instability.

Osmond-Clarke described with colour illustrations the precise steps of the Putti–Platt operation. **Adams** analysed the Royal Air Force experience of recurrent dislocation of the shoulder and showed the very small recurrence rate after both the Putti–Platt and the Bankart procedures. The paper discussed the pathology and stressed the frequency and importance of the humeral head defect. The principle topic of debate in this field is the treatment of recurrent anterior dislocation and we have included three further papers on different types of operation (**Rowe, Hovelius** and **Karadimas**) to present results on a large series and with a description of the procedure. The results would appear very similar and the type of repair performed seems to depend on the individual training of the surgeon and personal preference. The paper by **Leslie** has been included as the axillary incision avoids the ugly scar of the anterior approach.

Rowe discussed the management of the rare but difficult chronic unreduced dislocation. It was concluded that the overall prognosis for surgical treatment of the chronic unreduced dislocated shoulder is more favourable than previously reported.

Posterior dislocations are rare and still easily missed; the problems of diagnosis are discussed by **Nobel. McLaughlin** in a well known contribution distinguished between fixed and recurrent posterior subluxations of the shoulder and discussed their management.

Leffert has drawn attention to the generally favourable prognosis of brachial plexus lesions associated with closed injury in the region of the shoulder.

Acute Tears of the Rotator Cuff

The Classic

McLaughlin HL **Lesions of the musculotendinous cuff of the shoulder. I. The exposure and treatment of tears with retraction** J Bone Joint Surg 1944;42:31–51

Treatment

Bassett RW, Cofield RH **Acute tears of the rotator cuff – the timing of surgical repair** Clin Orthop 1983;175:18–24

Hawkins RJ **Surgical management of rotator cuff tears** In: Bateman JE, Welsh RP, ed. Surgery of the shoulder St. Louis, etc: CV Mosby 1984:161–166

Three papers on rotator cuff injuries have been included although these occur more commonly as a chronic lesion which is outside the scope of this book. **McLaughlin**'s paper is the classic and not as historical as the date of publication would now appear. There is a detailed description of the transacromial approach to the rotator cuff. **Bassett** discussed the indications and timing of repair of acute rotator cuff tears without a bony fragment. In patients who place high demands on their shoulders he advised early surgery where there is an acute injury and severe loss of function. **Hawkins** has presented a recent outlook on rotator cuff injuries based on over 100 rotator cuff reconstructions. Although the majority of such tears have been treated conservatively, we suspect there is a trend towards more aggressive early repair.

Fractures of the Proximal Humerus

Classification

Neer CS **Displaced proximal humeral fractures. Part I. Classification and evaluation** J Bone Joint Surg [Am] 1970;52-A:1077–1089

Treatment

Neer CS **Displaced proximal humeral fractures. Part II. Treatment of three-part and four-part displacement** J Bone Joint Surg [Am] 1970;52-A:1090–1103

Stableforth PG **Four-part fractures of the neck of the humerus** J Bone Joint Surg [Br] 1984;66-B:104–108

Young TB, Wallace WA **Conservative treatment of fractures and fracture dislocations of the upper end of the humerus** J Bone Joint Surg [Br] 1985;67-B:373–377

Epiphyseal Injuries

Baxter MP, Wiley JJ **Fractures of the proximal humeral epiphysis: their influence on humeral growth** J Bone Joint Surg [Br] 1986;68-B:570–573

Nerve Injury

Leffert RD, Seddon HJ **Infraclavicular brachial plexus injuries** J Bone Joint Surg [Br] 1965;47-B:9–22

The classic works on this subject are the two papers by **Neer,** based on a study of 300 cases. In the first he defined the traumatic anatomy of displaced fractures and proposed the classification that has been accepted by all subsequent authors. This classification described four major fragments of the proximal fracture and their potential displacement under the influence of muscle attachments. Both papers provide basic knowledge, are easy to read and well illustrated. Problems in treatment mainly relate to the management of the displaced three- and four-part fractures and the articles by **Neer** and **Stableforth** both indicate the difficulties experienced in obtaining a good result. The firm trend at the present time on this controversial subject is for operative treatment for these difficult injuries. In a prospective study of 49 patients **Stableforth** showed that reconstruction of the upper end of the humerus with insertion of a Neer prosthesis will usually restore comfort and function. However, the paper by **Young** is included as a contemporary series demonstrating that the majority of humeral neck fractures are relatively undisplaced and can be treated conservatively with a good or satisfactory result in 94% of cases six months from injury.

In children, the proximal end of the humerus demonstrates a remarkable capacity to remodel and an excellent result can follow a fracture with gross displacement. In **Baxter**'s article serial radiographs demonstrate the dramatic remodelling that can occur with growth and it is confirmed that open reduction is rarely indicated.

Leffert has drawn attention to the generally favourable prognosis of brachial plexus lesions associated with closed injury in the region of the shoulder. However, he noted the poor prognosis for isolated circumflex nerve injuries.

Fractures of the Shaft of the Humerus

Clinical Studies and Treatment

Klenerman L **Fracture of the shaft of the humerus** J Bone Joint Surg [Br] 1966; 48-B:105–111

Sarmiento A, Kinman PB, Galvin EG, Schmitt RH, Phillips JG **Functional bracing of fractures of the shaft of the humerus** J Bone Joint Surg [Am] 1977;59-A:596–601

Bell MJ, Beauchamp CG, Kellam JK, McMurtry RY **The results of plating humeral shaft fractures in patients with multiple injuries** J Bone Joint Surg [Br] 1985;67-B:293–296

Stern PJ, Mattingly DA, Pomeroy DL, Zenni EJ, Krieg JK **Intramedullary fixation of humeral shaft fractures** J Bone Joint Surg [Am] 1984;66-A:639–646

Complications

Pritchett JW **Delayed union of humeral shaft fractures treated by closed flexible intramedullary nailing** J Bone Joint Surg [Br] 1985;67-B:715–718

Holstein A **Fractures of the humerus with radial-nerve paralysis** J Bone Joint Surg [Am] 1963;45-A:1382–1388

Pollock FH, Drake D, Beauvill EG, Day L, Trafton PG **Treatment of radial neuropathy associated with fractures of the humerus** J Bone Joint Surg [Am] 1981;63-A:239–243

Bostman O, Bakalim G, Vainionpaa S, Wilppula E, Patiala A, Rokkanen P **Immediate radial nerve palsy complicating fractures of the shaft of the humerus: when is early exploration justified?** Injury 1985;16:499–502

Surgical Techniques

Henry AK **Approach to the whole back of the humeral shaft exposing from behind the neurovascular bundles of the arm** In: Extensile Exposure. 2nd edn. Edinburgh, etc: E & S Livingstone, 1970:15–25

Ruedi T, Von Hochstetter AHC, Schulmpf R **Section 4. Humeral shaft: antero-lateral approach.** pp 21–27 **Section 5. Humeral shaft: posterior approach.** pp 29–35 In: Surgical Approaches for Internal Fixation. Berlin, etc: Springer-Verlag, 1984

The accepted treatment for this injury is by one of several conservative methods and these are illustrated and justified by the figures in the articles by **Klenerman** and **Sarmiento**. The main indication for surgical treatment is the patient with multiple injuries. The paper by **Bell** and his colleagues gives an excellent account of their experience and of their satisfactory results. **Stern** discussed the use of intramedullary fixation in 70 fractures where closed treatment had failed or was considered inadequate; in these circumstances there was a significant morbidity and complications occurred in 67%.

Intramedullary fixation has been advocated for delayed union and **Pritchett**'s paper described the use of flexible nails introduced via the olecranon fossa, thus avoiding any significant impingement at the shoulder. Nine fractures healed out of a total of 10 without bone grafting. The management of associated radial nerve palsy is considered in three papers. **Holstein** considered that when paralysis of the radial nerve complicated a fracture of the shaft of the humerus, a specific situation exists. The fracture is spiral, in the distal third of the bone, and the distal fragment displaced proximally. Seven cases were described and open reduction recommended. **Pollock** noted a high incidence of complete recovery with conservative treatment and recommended exploration of the nerve at 4 months after injury if there was still no clinical or electro-myographic evidence of recovery. **Bostman** further debated this subject concluding that the need for early surgical exploration was more likely in the spiral or oblique fracture of the distal third of the shaft.

Henry and **Ruedi** provide excellent descriptions of the exposure of the humerus shaft and radial nerve. They are useful reminders even to the most experienced!

Fractures of the Distal Humerus in the Adult

Classification and Treatment

Brown RF, Morgan RG **Intercondylar "T" shaped fractures of the humerus. results in 10 cases treated by early mobilisation** J Bone Joint Surg [Br] 1971; 53-B:425–428

Jupite JB, Neff U, Holzach P, Allgower M **Intercondylar fractures of the humerus: an operative approach** J Bone Joint Surg [Am] 1985;67-A:226–239

Riseborough EH, Radin EL **Intercondylar "T" fractures of the humerus in adults. A comparison of operative and non-operative treatment in 29 cases** J Bone Joint Surg [Am] 1969;51-A:130–141

Zagorski JB, Jenning JJ, Burkhalter WE, Uribe JW **Comminuted intra-articular fractures of the distal humeral condyle** Clin Orthop 1986;202:197–204

The literature confirms the difficulties of management of these uncommon but often comminuted fractures with involvement of the articular surface of the elbow joint. **Brown** described the fair results that may be obtained by early mobilisation. The general trend of recent articles has been towards accurate open reduction, internal fixation and early movement. **Jupiter** from Basle described the Muller classification of these fractures and showed impressive radiographs of severe injuries. Detailed operative technique and results are given and appear to be excellent. The articles by **Riseborough** and later **Zagorski** both compare the results of conservative against surgical treatment in retrospective studies. There is some 17 years between their dates of publication and in that time the consensus of opinion has swung from traction to open reduction and fixation as the method of choice. In the more recent Zagorski article there is a good description of an interesting approach to the distal humerus.

Supracondylar Fractures of the Humerus in Children

Remodelling

Attenborough CG, **Remodelling of the humerus after supracondylar fractures in childhood** J Bone Joint Surg [Br] 1953;35-B:386–395

Charnley J **Supracondylar fractures of the humerus in children**. In: The closed treatment of common fractures 3rd edn Edinburgh, etc: E & S Livingstone, 1961:105–115

Methods of Treatment

Rang M **Supracondylar fractures** In: Children's fractures, 2nd edn Philadelphia: JB Lippincott, 1983:154–169

Worlock P **Supracondylar fractures of the humerus – assessment of cubitus varus by the Baumann angle** J Bone Joint Surg [Br] 1986;68-B:755–757

Piggot J, Graham HK, McCoy GF **Supracondylar fractures of the humerus in children: treatment by straight lateral traction** J Bone Joint Surg [Br] 1986; 68-B:577–583

Flynn JC, Matthews JG, Benoit RL **Blind pinning of displaced supracondylar fractures of the humerus in children – 16 years experience with long-term follow-up** J Bone Joint Surg [Am] 1974;56-A:263–272

Weiland AJ, Meye S, Tolo VT, Berg HL, Mueller J **Surgical treatment of displaced supracondylar fractures of the humerus in children – an analysis of 52 cases followed for 5–15 years** J Bone Joint Surg [Am] 1978;60-A:657–661

Pirone AM, Graham HK, Krajbich JI **Management of displaced extension-type supracondylar fractures of the humerus in children** J Bone Joint Surg [Am] 1988;70-A:641–650

Treatment of Cubitus Varus

Bellemore MC, Barrett IR, Middleton RWD, Scougall JS, Whiteway DW **Supracondylar osteotomy of the humerus for correction of cubitus varus** J Bone Joint Surg [Br] 1984;66-B:566–572

Volkmann's Contracture

Holden CEA **The pathology and prevention of Volkmann's contracture** J Bone Joint Surg [Br] 1979;61-B:296–300

Mubarak SJ, Carroll NC **Volkmann's contracture in children: aetiology and prevention** J Bone Joint Surg [Br] 1979;61-B:285–293

Seddon Sir HJ **Volkmann's contracture: treatment by excision of the infarct** J Bone Joint Surg [Br] 1956;38-B:152–174

The management of a displaced supracondylar fracture in a child is a controversial and difficult subject and may cause anxiety even to the experienced surgeon. The various possible methods of standard treatment are described by **Rang** and the importance of remodelling with growth by both **Attenborough** and **Charnley**.

There would appear still to be uncertainty and debate as to the relative importance of persistent medial tilting and medial rotation, in the production of late cubitus varus deformity. Possibly this may be due to the difficulty of accurate radiological assessment of the reduced position after manipulative reduction. **Worlock** has recently attempted to remedy this lack of knowledge by careful measurement of the Baumann angle in patients treated by overhead skeletal traction. **Piggot** described the results of 98 displaced supracondylar fractures with neurovascular problems, gross swelling or instability treated by straight lateral traction. At follow-up cubitus varus was present in only four children. Changing attitudes to the management of these injuries is also reflected by the use of manipulative reduction and blind pinning by **Flynn**. Older orthopaedic surgeons have believed and taught that open reduction and internal fixation of this fracture is very seldom required since there is an alleged certainty of residual stiffness of the joint. **Weiland** has described a series of 52 cases followed from 5 to 15 years with good results. **Flynn**'s paper included a concise summary of the well recognised vascular and neurological complications of this injury. Results of treatment in 230 patients by four different methods have been recently compared by **Pirone**. The best results were achieved by percutaneous K-wire fixation and this is recommended. An arresting conclusion was that closed reduction and a plaster cast gave a lower percentage of excellent results. **Bellemore** described the technique and results of supracondylar osteotomy for the correction of cubitus varus.

Reference to Volkmann's contracture has been included since distal ischaemia frequently causes anxiety during early treatment. **Holden** discussed the significance of severe persistent pain after manipulation. **Mubarak** stressed the importance and indications for early fasciotomy. **Seddon** has been included to provide basic knowledge on the pathology of Volkmann's contracture.

Epiphyseal Injuries of the Distal Humerus

Lateral Condyle

Jakob R, Fowles JV, Rang M, Kassab MT **Observations concerning fractures of the lateral humeral condyle in children** J Bone Joint Surg [Br] 1975; 57-B:430–436

Rang M **Fractures of the lateral condyle** In: Children's fractures, 2nd edn Philadelphia, etc: JB Lippincott, 1983:173–179

Papavasiliou VA, Beslikas TA **Fractures of the lateral humeral condyle in children – an analysis of 39 cases** Injury 1985;16:364–366

Jeffery CC **Non-union of the epiphysis of the lateral condyle of the humerus** J Bone Joint Surg [Br] 1958;40-B:396–405

Epiphyseal injuries around the elbow can be difficult to diagnose and treat correctly. **Jakob** considered that in fractures of the lateral humeral condyle in children, the mechanism of injury is a violent varus force with the elbow in extension. The major problem of a neglected fracture is tardy ulnar palsy. **Rang** stated that undisplaced fractures healed well with cast immobilisation but internal fixation is essential if there is any doubt that an accurate reduction has been achieved. The results of treatment of 39 cases 3 to 12 years after injury were described by **Papavasiliou**. Mal-union and non-union occurred only in patients who were treated without operation. The paper by **Jeffrey** contained some cautionary radiographs illustrating the circumstances in which non-union occurred, its prevention and treatment. There were 13 cases of non-union and 10 of these followed minor lateral subluxation of the epiphysis.

Medial Epicondyle

Papavasiliou VA **Fracture-separation of the medial epicondylar epiphysis of the elbow joint** Clin Orthop 1982;171:172–174

The injury of the medial epicondyle is common and should be usually treated conservatively. **Papavasiliou**'s paper reviewed 91 cases with a long follow-up and contained sound advice on avoiding problems, particularly that of the fragment trapped within the elbow joint.

Dislocations of the Elbow

Hassman GC, Brunn F, Neer CS **Recurrent dislocation of the elbow** J Bone Joint Surg [Am] 1975;57-A:1080–1084

Krishnamoorthy S, Bose K, Wong KP **Treatment of old unreduced dislocation of the elbow** Injury 1976;8:39–42

Treatment and results of simple elbow dislocation provoke little controversy. We have, however, included a paper on each of two unusual but difficult problems. The study by **Hassman** is of only four cases and included a review of the literature but the problem of recurrent dislocation is clearly described and lateral repair recommended. The work by **Krishnamoorthy** on late presentation of elbow dislocation is from Singapore and presented a large experience of a rare problem. The surgical technique is well described and the results and follow-up are impressive.

Fractures of the Radial Head in the Adult

The Classic

Radin EL, Riseborough EJ **Fractures of the radial head. A review of 88 cases and analysis of the indications for excision of the radial head and non-operative treatment.** J Bone Joint Surg [Am] 1966;48-A:1055–1064

Excision

Coleman DA, Blair WF, Shurr D **Resection of the radial head for fracture of the radial head** J Bone Joint Surg [Am] 1987;69-A:385–392

Mikic ZD, Vukadinovic SV **Late results in fractures of the radial head treated by excision** Clin Orthop 1983;181:220–228

Internal Fixation

Shmueli G, Herold HZ **Compression screwing of displaced fractures of the head of the radius** J Bone Joint Surg [Br] 1981;63-B:535–538

Silastic Replacement

Morrey BF, Askew L, Chao EY **Silastic prosthetic replacement for the radial head** J Bone Joint Surg [Am] 1981;63-A:454–458

Mackay I, Fitzgerald B, Miller JH **Silastic replacement of the head of the radius in trauma** J Bone Joint Surg [Br] 1979;61-B:494–497

Radin studied 88 patients observed for at least two years after injury. A realistic description is presented of the outcome in the different types of fracture. The principle subject of controversy is the treatment of displaced segmental fractures. A careful analysis is presented of the indications and results of conservative treatment versus excision of the radial head. Displaced fractures involving less than two-thirds of the radial head should be treated by early movement; where the displaced fracture involved more then two-thirds of the radial head, early total excision should be performed.

The papers by **Coleman** and **Mikic** reflect the continuing discussion and present widely differing results of excision of the head of the radius.

Shmueli advocated open reduction and insertion of a compression screw in selected cases with a displaced fracture. Rigid fixation allowed immediate mobilisation.

The paper by **Morrey** described experience and results with silastic replacement for the radial head in 17 patients. There were five failures and he concluded that the indications for replacement were limited. Long-term results are required. The paper by **Mackay** has been included since a prosthesis was particularly effective in those patients with an associated posterior dislocation of the elbow and provided increased stability.

Fractures of the Head and Neck of the Radius in Children

Jeffery CC **Fractures of the head of the radius in children** J Bone Joint Surg [Br] 1950;32-B:314–324

Jones ERL, Esah M **Displaced fractures of the neck of the radius in children** J Bone Joint Surg [Br] 1971;53-B:429–439

Newman JH **Displaced radial neck fractures in children** Injury 1977;9:114–121

Jeffery discussed the mechanism of injury and treatment of 24 cases and especially described and illustrated the lateral tilting and technique of manipulative reduction. **Jones** described experience with 34 cases and concluded that all fractures, whatever the age of the child, with angular displacement exceeding 15 degrees need accurate reduction. Closed reduction is not easy; fractures which are unstable require internal fixation with Kirschner wires. **Newman** studied a group of 48 children, described five patterns of radial neck injury and especially stressed the occurrence of complications including avascular necrosis and radio-ulnar synostosis. He concluded that treatment of these fractures should be by closed means whenever possible.

Fractures of the Olecranon

Holdsworth BJ, Mossad MM **Elbow function following tension band fixation of displaced fractures of the olecranon** Injury 1984;16:182–187

Deliyannis SN **Comminuted fractures of the olecranon treated by the Weber–Vasey technique** Injury 1973;5:19–24

Fyfe IS, Mossad MM, Holdsworth BJ **Methods of fixation of olecranon fractures – an experimental mechanical study** J Bone Joint Surg [Br] 1985; 67-B:367–372

Gartsman GM, Sculco TP, Otis JC **Operative treatment of olecranon fractures – excision or open reduction with internal fixation** J Bone Joint Surg [Am] 1981; 63-A:718–721

This common injury is usually treated by means of a tension band wire with 85% good results as shown by **Holdsworth**. **Deliyannis** showed that the method is applicable in comminuted fractures which are usually considered the most difficult to treat. A number of other methods of fixation have been used and a paper on the biomechanics of fixation by **Fyfe** compared the rigidity of the more commonly used techniques. Tension band wiring with two tightening knots allowed least movement even at higher loads. A single cancellous screw gave the most erratic results. A paper by **Gartsman** has been included which compared the results of excision with internal fixation. Good results were claimed for excision and the study provided a reminder that excision has been a popular method of treatment in the past and is an option worthy of consideration in some exceptional circumstances.

Fractures of the Shaft of the Radius and Ulna in the Adult

Clinical Studies

Anderson LD, Sisk TD, Tooms RE, Park WI **Compression-plate fixation in acute diaphyseal fractures of the radius and ulna** J Bone Joint Surg [Am] 1975; 57-A:287–297

Hadden WA, Reschauer R, Seggl W **Results of AO plate fixation of forearm shaft fractures in adults** Injury 1983;15:44–52

Corea JR, Brakenbury PH, Blakemore ME **The treatment of isolated fractures of the ulna shaft in adults** Injury 1980;12:365–370

Brakenbury PH, Corea JR, Blakemore ME **Non-union of the isolated fracture of the ulna shaft in adults** Injury 1980;12:371–375

Hidaka S, Gustilo RB **Refracture of bones of the forearm after plate removal** J Bone Joint Surg [Am] 1984;66-A:1241–1243

Surgical Technique

Henry AK **The front of the forearm. The back of the forearm**. In: Extensile exposure 2nd edn Edinburgh: E & S Livingstone, 1970:94–105, 111–115

Ruedi T, von Hochstetter AHC, Schulmpf R **Radial shaft: dorsolateral approach**. In: Surgical approaches for the internal fixation Berlin, etc: Springer-Verlag, 1984:57–61

In the paper from the Campbell Clinic **Anderson** presented a review of the results of treatment of 330 acute fractures with an impressive rate of union of 97%. Details of their surgical technique are clearly described and complications discussed. **Hadden** described the treatment of 111 fractures by the AO method and performed by 18 different surgeons. There was a similar successful rate of union but a higher incidence of infection (6 cases). This method of treatment led to excellent results in a majority of patients but was associated with serious complications in a minority (non-union in seven). There were problems of cross-union in those who had a head injury. The two papers by **Corea** and **Brackenbury** discussed the management of 254 cases of isolated fracture of the shaft of the ulna. The indications for conservative and operative treatment are discussed and a plan of management is proposed. In those treated conservatively, they advocated the technique of functional bracing as described by Sarmiento (J Bone Joint Surg [Br] 1976;58-A:1104–1107). The second paper studied the possible cause of non-union of the ulna in 21 patients. **Hidaka** examined the problem of re-fracture after plate removal and noted that this occurred in 7 out of 32 cases. They discussed the possible causes of re-fracture after compression plating and recommended that a plate should not be removed before one year after application.

A detailed knowledge of operative exposure of the forearm bones is essential and reference is therefore included to the classical descriptions by **Henry** and **Ruedi**.

Fractures of the Shaft of the Radius and Ulna in Children

Clinical Studies

Rang M **The radius and ulna** In: Children's fractures, 2nd edn Philadelphia, etc: JB Lippincott, 1983:197–215

Fuller DJ, McCullough CJ **Mal-united fractures of the forearm in children** J Bone Joint Surg [Br] 1982;64-B:364–367

Nielsen AB, Simonsen O **Displaced forearm fractures in children treated with AO plates** Injury 1984;15:393–396

Volkmann's Contracture

Holden CEA **The pathology and prevention of Volkmann's contracture** J Bone Joint Surg [Br] 1979;61-B:296–300

Greenstick and complete fractures of the radius and ulna in children are usually treated by manipulative reduction and immobilisation and **Rang** discussed the principles of management, details of technique and the importance of remodelling. Remodelling does not correct rotation in older children. Mal-union can lead to permanent disability. The capacity of the radius and ulna to remodel spontaneously after mal-union was studied carefully by **Fuller** in 49 children. Mal-union of the distal third of the radius and ulna will remodel satisfactorily providing the child is less than 14 years of age. Gross mal-union of the mid-shaft of the radius and ulna will spontaneously correct in an infant but little useful correction of deformity can be anticipated in these fractures when the child is aged eight or more. A decision of acceptance of the position after manipulation, or alternatively, operative fixation is often not easy. **Nielsen** discussed the circumstances in which operative fixation was performed in 43 fractures.

Holden's paper is included to remind the reader of the vital importance of severe pain after these injuries since it may indicate ischaemia and demand urgent treatment.

Monteggia and Galeazzi Fractures

The Classic

Evans EM **Pronation injuries of the forearm with special reference to the anterior Monteggia fracture** J Bone Joint Surg [Br] 1949;31-B:578–588

Clinical Studies

Boyd HB, Boales JC **The Monteggia lesion – a review of 159 cases** Clin Orthop 1969;66:94–100

Letts M, Locht R, Weins J **Monteggia fracture-dislocations in children** J Bone Joint Surg [Br] 1985;67-B:724–727

Wiley JJ, Galey JP **Monteggia injuries in children** J Bone Joint Surg [Br] 1985; 67-B:728–731

Reckling FW **Unstable fracture-dislocations of the forearm (Monteggia and Galeazzi lesions)** J Bone Joint Surg [Am] 1982;64-A:857–863

Mikic ZD **Galeazzi fracture-dislocations** J Bone Joint Surg [Am]1975;57-A: 1071–1080

Evans in 1949 discussed the possible mechanism of injury based on experimental work on post-mortem specimens. He concluded that anterior dislocation of the head of the radius with or without fracture of the ulna is a forced pronation injury and that full supination is essential for reduction.

Boyd reviewed 159 cases treated at the Campbell Clinic and recommended stable internal fixation of the ulna and, rarely, if reduction of the head of the radius is incomplete, reconstruction of the annular ligament. The papers by **Letts** and **Wiley** have been included since they provide information on the diagnosis and management of the Monteggia injury in 79 children. In the paper by **Letts**, a new classification is proposed while **Wiley** used the Bado classification. Closed reduction was successful and recommended in both contributions. Open reduction was required only for older children or when treatment was begun late. **Reckling** studied a series of 49 Monteggia and 47 Galeazzi lesions over a 25-year period. In all of the children either closed or open reduction yielded good results but those in the adult varied. The management of each type of injury is outlined using the Bado classification. The results of closed reduction of the classic Galeazzi fractures in the adults were not good due to mal-union. Open reduction and internal fixation of the fractured radius with immobilisation in supination obtained good results. **Mikic** studied 127 patients and both **Reckling** and **Mikic** stressed the inherent instability and problems of management of some of these difficult injuries in the adult.

Colles' Fracture

The Classic

Charnley J **The Colles' fracture.** In: The closed treatment of common fractures 3rd edn Edinburgh, etc: E & S Livingstone, 1961:128–142

Conservative Treatment

Stewart HD, Innes AR, Burke FD **Functional cast-bracing for Colles' fractures. A comparison between cast-bracing and conventional plaster casts** J Bone Joint Surg [Br] 1984;66-B:749–753

McQueen MM, MacLaren A, Chalmers J **The value of re-manipulating Colles' fractures** J Bone Joint Surg [Br] 1986;68-B:232–233

Dias JJ, Wray CC, Jones JM, Gregg PJ **The value of early mobilisation in the treatment of Colles' fractures** J Bone Joint Surg [Br] 1987;69-B:463–467

Surgical Treatment

Jenkins NH, Jones DG, Johnson SR, Mintowt-Czyz WJ **External fixation of Colles' fractures – an anatomical study** J Bone Joint Surg [Br] 1987;69-B: 207–211

Weber SC, Szabo RM **Severely comminuted distal radial fracture as an unsolved problem. Complications associated with external fixation and pins and plaster techniques.** J Hand Surgery [Am] 1986;11-A:157–165

Melone CP **Articular fractures of the distal radius** Orthop Clin North Am 1984;15:217–236

Complications

Cooney WP, Dobyns JH, Linscheid RL **Complications of Colles' fractures** J Bone Joint Surg [Am] 1980;62-A:613–619

Charnley's chapter covers the anatomy of Colles' fracture and the practical technique of conservative management.

Stewart studied three different methods of immobilisation and concluded that the anatomical result was not influenced by the method of immobilisation but was related to the accuracy of reduction. Loss of position in a brace was no greater than in plaster. The functional result at three months was, however, related to the severity of the initial displacement. **McQueen** concluded that in patients over the age of 60 re-manipulation failed to achieve a lasting improvement and therefore such patients did not benefit from this procedure. **Dias** reported a study of a randomised prospective trial and concluded that early wrist movement hastened functional recovery. The bony deformity, which recurred irrespective of the method of treatment, was not adversely affected by early mobilisation.

The literature in the last decade reflects less acceptance of bad results in these injuries, especially in younger patients. There has therefore been a trend towards external fixation, reported in detail by both **Jenkins** and **Weber**. **Jenkins** found that the external fixator was more effective in holding the manipulated position and the radiological loss of position during fracture union was minimal. **Weber** drew attention to the unsolved problem of the severe comminuted fracture of the distal radius and the complications associated with external fixation and pin and plaster techniques. The Frykman classification (Acta Orthop Scand 1967; Suppl 108) is discussed. External fixation maintained radial length but did not correct the dorsal tilt or the "die-punch" fragment involving the joint. The complication rate for younger, often multiply injured patients was high. **Melone** described four types of articular fracture and noted the hallmark of the unstable fracture is comminution of both the posterior and anterior cortices of the radius (die-punch fracture).

Cooney's paper reviewed 565 distal radial fractures and reported a 31% complication rate involving neuropathy, arthritis, mal-union and tendon ruptures. However, this complication rate may be higher than other reports since 46% of patients reviewed were referred from other centres for management.

Smith's Fracture

Clinical Studies

Thomas FB **Reduction of Smith's fracture** J Bone Joint Surg [Br] 1957; 39-B:463–471

Ellis J **Smith's and Barton's fractures – a method of treatment** J Bone Joint Surg [Br] 1965;47-B:724–727

Fuller DJ **The Ellis plate operation for Smith's fracture** J Bone Joint Surg [Br] 1973;55-B:173–178

Surgical Technique

Muller ME, Allgower M, Schneider R, Willenegger H **Manual of internal fixation**, 2nd edn Berlin,etc: Springer-Verlag, 1979:194–197

In 1957, **Thomas** described three types of Smith's fracture and suggested that the majority of these fractures are caused by pronation injury. Treatment recommended was therefore reduction and immobilisation in a plaster cast with the elbow included and the forearm supinated. **Ellis** concisely described the history of the fractures ascribed to Smith and Barton and outlined the operative treatment for fixation of these fractures with an anterior buttress plate. **Fuller** reviewed 31 patients who were treated for a Smith's fracture by the Ellis plate. Open reduction and plate fixation was particularly indicated in those patients with an anterior marginal fracture and subluxation forwards of the carpus. **Muller** described and illustrated the operative technique using an AO plate.

Section 3
The Hand

Primary Treatment of the Acutely Injured Hand

The Classic

James JIP **Assessment and management of the injured hand** Hand 1970;2: 97–105

Primary Treatment

Semple C **Primary treatment of the acutely injured hand.** In: Birch R, Brooks D ed. The hand. 4th edn (Rob and Smith's operative surgery) London, etc: Butterworth, 1984:61–70

Brown PW **Open injuries of the hand.** In: Green DP ed. Operative hand surgery. Vol. 2, 2nd edn Edinburgh, etc: Churchill Livingstone, 1988:1619–1653

Skin Cover

Harrison SH **Principles of skin replacement in the hand** Hand 1970;2: 106–111

Cobbett JR **The free graft** Hand 1970;2:112–115

Kinmonth MH **The use of skin flaps in hand injuries** Hand 1970;2:116–118

Evans DM **The management of the skin in injuries of the hand.** In: Lamb DW, Hooper G, Kuczynski K ed. The practice of hand surgery. 2nd edn Oxford: Blackwell Scientific Publications, 1989:121–149

Lister GD, McGregor IA, Jackson IT **The groin flap in hand injuries** Injury 1972;4:229–239

Freedlander E, Dickson WA, McGrouther DA **Present role of the groin flap in hand trauma in the light of a long-term review** J Hand Surg [Br] 1986; 11-B:187–190

Lister G, Scheker L **Emergency free flaps to the upper extremity** J Hand Surg [Am] 1988;13-A:22–28

James stressed that there are three causes of stiffness in the injured hand after injury: infection, faulty joint position and oedema. Methods of prevention of joint stiffness are discussed and the method of splintage and bandaging to avoid the stiffness illustrated.

Semple described the various types of injury of the hand and essential primary management, including details of operative treatment of the wound and fractures and dislocations. **Brown** discussed the order of priority for open wound management in the injured hand. Debridement, the achievement of skeletal stability and wound closure are debated. There are specific sections discussing the management of degloving, amputation and mangling.

The papers by **Harrison**, **Cobbett** and **Kinmonth** were published as part of a symposium in 1970. The knowledge presented is basic but it has been included to remind the reader of principles. **Cobbett** stressed that primary split skin cover should always be used unless the surgeon has special experience, or there is an open joint or tendon sheath.

Evans has summarised the present approach to skin cover in the injured hand. Split thickness skin grafts are still considered the safest and simplest free grafts after injury. Detailed technique is described. The use of more complicated cross-finger, thenar and groin flaps are discussed and, finally, there is a section on micro-vascular free flaps. Early and appropriate referral for major skin loss is stressed.

The basis of the groin flap for severe hand injuries was described by **Lister** and **Freedlander** discussed the merits and disadvantages of this flap based on experience of 73 cases. Many severely injured hands have been successfully reconstructed by the use of the groin flap.

A paper by **Lister** on emergency free flaps has been included to indicate recent trends with successful micro-vascular transfer. Although not usually the direct concern of the orthopaedic surgeon, it is suggested that he should be aware of these developments.

Anaesthesia in Hand Surgery

Chan KM, Ma GFY, Chow YN, Leung PC **Intravenous regional anaesthesia in hand surgery – experience with 632 cases** Hand 1981;13:192–198

Ramamurthy S **Anaesthesia**. In: Green DP, ed. Operative hand surgery. 2nd edn, Vol 1. Edinburgh, etc: Churchill Livingstone, 1988:27–60

Raggi RP **Balanced regional anaesthesia for hand surgery** Orthop Clin North Am 1986;17:473–482

Chan has presented a large experience of 632 cases of intravenous regional anaesthesia for hand surgery with a practical guide to the steps involved and the avoidance of complications. The technique is safe, simple and efficient. **Ramamurthy** has described the precise technique with illustrations of the various types of regional block anaesthesia which may be necessary for the hand. Controversies in hand anaesthesia revolve around general versus regional, patient selection, technique and agents and these have recently been debated by **Raggi**.

Fractures of the Scaphoid

The Classic

London PS **The broken scaphoid** J Bone Joint Surg [Br] 1961;43-B:237–244

Natural History and Conservative Management

Leslie I J, Dickson RA **The fractured carpal scaphoid** J Bone Joint Surg [Br] 1984;66-B:225–230

Non-Union

Mack GR, Bosse MJ, Gelberman RH, Yu E **The natural history of scaphoid non-union** J Bone Joint Surg [Am] 1984;66-A:504–509

Surgical Treatment

Herbert TJ, Fisher WE **Management of the fractured scaphoid using a new bone screw** J Bone Joint Surg [Br] 1984;66-B:114–123

Dooley BJ **Inlay bone grafting for non-union of the scaphoid by the anterior approach** J Bone Joint Surg [Br] 1968;50-B:102–109

Herbert TJ **Scaphoid fractures: operative treatment.** In: Barton NJ, ed. Fractures of the hand and wrist Edinburgh, etc: Churchill Livingstone, 1988: 220–235

London's paper in 1961 is included since 95% of all fractures of the scaphoid under a month old united with "proper" treatment. **Leslie** investigated the natural history of these injuries based on a study of 222 consecutive patients and confirmed that a union rate of 95% could be achieved using standard immobilisation in a plaster cast.

Mack showed that very few patients with non-union of the scaphoid were free of degenerative arthritis ten years after injury and they recommend that all displaced scaphoid fractures should be reduced and treated by a bone graft. Where the fresh fracture is appreciably displaced, or where delayed or non-union occurs, treatment is never easy.

The relatively new contribution by **Herbert** described the use of a bone screw and the results achieved for both fresh fractures and those with delayed or non-union may well be a considerable advance. **Dooley**'s paper and the adjacent one by Mulder discussed the results of both grafting of the scaphoid by the anterior approach originally described by Russe. It is possible that this method of treatment may have been superseded by the use of Herbert's screw with a bone graft but is included since the subject is controversial. The reader should be aware of this technique and the good results that can be achieved. A further recent paper by **Herbert** outlined the continuing debate on the likely result of conventional treatment for fresh fractures and on the need for reconstructive surgery of the carpus in non-union.

Dislocations of the Carpus

Panting AL, Lamb DW, Noble J, Haw CS **Dislocations of the lunate with and without fracture of the scaphoid** J Bone Joint Surg [Br] 1984;66-B:391–395

Green DP, O'Brien ET **Open reduction of carpal dislocations: indications and operative technique** J Hand Surg [Am] 1978;3-A:250–265

Cooney WP, Bussey R, Dobyns JH, Linscheid RL **Difficult wrist fractures. Perilunate fracture-dislocations of the wrist** Clin Orthop 1987;214:136–147

Carpal dislocations are rare, major and complex injuries. **Green** presented a classification and plan of management based on the belief that lunate and perilunate dislocations are different stages of the same injury. Displacement may be either volar or dorsal. It is vital to obtain and maintain excellent reduction, if necessary by open reduction and internal fixation. **Panting** noted that most patients with a simple dislocation of the lunate had satisfactory results at follow-up of $3^1/_2$ years. Immediate percutaneous wire fixation of the reduced scaphoid, whether fractured or not, is recommended for maintenance of stability. **Green** reported experience with a relatively large series of 49 cases of carpal dislocation. In trans-scaphoid perilunate dislocations, failure to reduce the scaphoid anatomically is an indication for primary open reduction. **Cooney** recently described the results of primary open reduction of 21 patients with carpal fracture-dislocations of the wrist. Avascular necrosis of either the scaphoid or the lunate occurred in 13.

Carpal Instability

Fisk GR **The wrist** J Bone Joint Surg [Br] 1984;66-B:396–407

Linscheid RL, Dobyns JH, Beabout EW, Bryan RS **Traumatic instability of the wrist. Diagnosis, classification and pathomechanics** J Bone Joint Surg [Am] 1972;54-A:1612–1632

Taleisnik J **Post-traumatic carpal instability** Clin Orthop 1980;149:73–82

In view of the increasing interest, three papers have been included on the subject of carpal instability. **Fisk** presented a thoughtful review on the general subject of the wrist and the causes, diagnosis and treatment of carpal instability are considered. He stressed that the lunate is the "lynch pin" of the wrist. **Linscheid** described two types of post-traumatic instability: dorsal and volar, depending essentially on the relation of the lunate to the radius in the lateral view. **Taleisnik** proposed a classification of the subtle forms of this condition exclusive of the more severe fractures, dislocations and fracture-dislocations.

Fractures of the Hand

Review Article

Barton NJ **Fractures of the hand** J Bone Joint Surg [Br] 1984;66-B:159–167

Bennett's Fracture

Pollen AG **The conservative treatment of Bennett's fracture subluxation of the thumb metacarpal** J Bone Joint Surg [Br] 1968;50-B:91–101

Cannon SR, Dowd GSE, Williams DH, Scott JM **A long-term study following Bennett's fracture** J Hand Surg [Br] 1986;11-B:426–431

Foster RJ, Hastings H **Treatment of Bennett, Rolando and vertical intra-articular trapezial fractures** Clin Orthop 1987;214:121–129

Fractures of the Metacarpals

Lamb DW **Fractures of the neck and shaft of the metacarpals**. In: Barton NJ, ed. Fractures of the hand and wrist Edinburgh, etc: Churchill Livingstone, 1988: 108–119

In the article by **Barton**, a concise review is presented on the reduction, retention and rehabilitation of fractures of the hand with special reference to principles and the use of conservative and operative treatment.

Pollen reviewed 31 patients treated by manipulation and a carefully moulded plaster cast as previously described by Charnley. Twenty-nine were successfully treated in this way and operation was required in only two. In a study of 25 patients, reviewed for a mean of nine years, **Cannon** showed that there was little evidence that imperfect reduction leads to significant symptomatic arthritis in the long term. The operative technique has been described in detail by **Foster**.

The treatment of fractures of the metacarpal bones is usually considered to be uncontroversial, especially in the majority which are stable. However, **Lamb** has drawn attention to the prevention of a rotary deformity and to the trend towards internal fixation with Kirchner wires for unstable fractures, particularly when multiple or associated with open injuries or skin loss.

Fractures of the Phalanges

James JIP **Fractures of the shafts of the phalanges: conservative treatment** In: Barton NJ, ed. Fractures of the hand and wrist Edinburgh, etc: Churchill Livingstone, 1988:22–31

Belsky MR, Eaton RG **Fractures of the shafts of the phalanges: percutaneous wire fixation** In: Barton NJ, ed. Fractures of the hand and wrist Edinburgh, etc: Churchill Livingstone, 1988:41–46

Kutz JE, Ruff ME **Fractures of the shafts of the phalanges: open reduction and internal fixation** In: Barton NJ, ed. Fractures of the hand and wrist Edinburgh, etc: Churchill Livingstone, 1988:47–54

Mulligan PJ **Comminuted fractures** In: Barton NJ, ed. Fractures of the hand and wrist Edinburgh, etc: Churchill Livingstone, 1988:74–86

There are no trivial injuries of the hand, least of all, a fractured finger. There is now increased awareness of the importance of skill and care in the management of fractures of the phalanges, particularly those that are displaced and this is therefore reflected in the short chapters chosen in this section. **James** has described in detail the method of splintage which he has advocated for the maintenance of reduction of phalangeal fractures and later, the restoration of function and avoidance of a stiff finger. There is still considerable controversy concerning the indications for percutaneous wire fixation and open reduction of the displaced fracture and this is indicated by **Belsky** and **Kutz**. **Mulligan** has stressed the importance of crush injuries which may lead to severe oedema and stiffness. On many occasions, splintage is not possible and hence, stabilisation is achieved by various methods of fixation including external fixation.

Operative Technique

Barton NJ **Operative treatment of fractures of the hand** In: Birch R, Brooks D, ed. The Hand. 4th edn. (Rob and Smith's Operative Surgery) London: Butterworth, 1984:184–195

Heim U, Pfeiffer KM **The hand** In: Internal fixation of small fractures. Technique recommended by the AO-ASIF Group. 3rd edn Berlin, etc: Springer-Verlag, 1988:179–246

Precise technique for operative treatment of fractures of the hand is described by **Barton**. This is further amplified by the description of the AO technique with many illustrations in the small fragment set manual by **Heim**.

Dislocations and Ligament Injuries in the Digits

The Proximal Interphalangeal Joint

Kuczynski K **The proximal interphalangeal joint. Anatomy and causes of stiffness in the fingers** J Bone Joint Surg [Br] 1968;50-B:656–663

Benke GJ, Stableforth PG **Injuries of the proximal interphalangeal joint of the fingers** Hand 1979;11:263–268

Dray GJ, Eaton RG **Dislocations and ligament injuries in the digits. The PIP joint** In: Green DP, ed. Operative hand surgery, 2nd edn, Vol.1 Edinburgh, etc: Churchill Livingstone, 1988:777–786

One of the most common and more serious problems of the injured finger is stiffness of the proximal interphalangeal joint either in flexion or, more rarely, in extension. **Kuczynski** has described the anatomy and discussed the causes of stiffness both in extension and flexion. If immobilisation of the proximal interphalangeal joint cannot be avoided, it should be for as short a period as possible. **Benke** studied the results of treatment of 96 injured proximal interphalangeal joints. The injuries are somewhat less common than is suggested in the literature. Ninety-five per cent excellent or good results occurred with hyperextension injuries without dislocation. At least 30% bad results occurred with dislocations and fracture-dislocations. The principle problem was stiffness with marked fixed flexion and loss of flexion. **Dray** divided acute dorsal dislocations into three types: (I) hyperextension, (II) dorsal dislocation and (III) fracture dislocation. The pathology was discussed with emphasis on damage to the volar plate. Operative treatment was necessary for unstable fracture dislocation. A dynamic extension splint is illustrated which permits active motion, thus reducing joint stiffness.

The Thumb Metacarpophalangeal Joint

Stenner B **Displacement of the ruptured ulnar collateral ligament of the metacarpophalangeal joint of the thumb. A clinical and anatomical study.** J Bone Joint Surg [Br] 1962;44-B:869–879

Lamb DW, Abernethy PJ, Fragiadakis E **Injuries of the metacarpophalangeal joint of the thumb** Hand 1971;3:164–168

Smith RJ **Post-traumatic instability of the metacarpophalangeal joint of the thumb** J Bone Joint Surg [Am] 1977;59-A:14–21

Osterman AL, Hayken GD, Bora FWM **A quantitative evaluation of thumb function after ulnar collateral repair and reconstruction** J Trauma 1981; 21:854–861

Stenner B **Repair of the ulnar collateral ligament of the thumb with and without chip fractures** In: Birch R, Brooks D, ed. The Hand. 4th edn. (Rob and Smith's Operative Surgery) London, etc: Butterworth, 1983;196–199

The classical paper by **Stenner** described the pathological anatomy of total rupture of the ulnar collateral ligament of the metacarpophalangeal joint of the thumb. The distally ruptured ligament retracts and the adductor aponeurosis becomes interposed between the ruptured ends adjacent to the phalanx. **Lamb** reviewed experience with 50 patients. In 15 of the 18 cases with instability, where operation was carried out within a week of injury, the displacement described by **Stenner** was confirmed. In one-third there was a delay in treatment of over one month. **Smith** noted instability on the radial side of the joint in one-quarter of a large series and in some there was volar subluxation. Early surgical treatment was recommended for all patients with instability greater than 45 degrees. **Osterman** described objective criteria for evaluation of results of surgical repair. If the diagnosis was made late, more than a few weeks after injury, treatment recommended was reconstruction or arthrodesis. **Stenner** has described and illustrated his recommended operative technique.

Flexor Tendon Injuries

Historical Review

Pulvertaft RG **Tendon grafts for flexor tendon injuries in the fingers and thumb. A study of technique and results** J Bone Joint Surg [Br] 1956; 38-B:175–194

Verdan CE **Half a century of flexor-tendon surgery. Current status and changing philosophies** J Bone Joint Surg [Am] 1972;54-A:472–491

Biology

Matthews P, Richards HJ **Factors in the adherence of flexor tendon after repair: an experimental study in the rabbit** J Bone Joint Surg [Br] 1976; 58-B:230–236

Over 30 years ago, **Pulvertaft** published a classical paper describing his remarkable results of 149 consecutive cases of flexor tendon grafting. Detailed technique is described. **Verdan**'s paper provided a historical perspective to flexor tendon surgery. He summarised advances that have been made in the knowledge of functional and pathological anatomy together with clinical experience. **Matthews** described an experimental study on the production of adhesions and referred to the classical work of Potenza. Splintage, suture and excision of the tendon sheath are all responsible in varying degrees for the adhesions that occur after tendon repair.

Clinical Aspects

Kleinert HE, Mears A **In quest of the solution to severed flexor tendons** Clin Orthop 1974;104:23–29

Lister GD, Kleinert HE, Kutz JE, Atasoy E **Primary flexor tendon repair followed by immediate controlled mobilisation** J Hand Surg 1977;2:441–451

Tubiana R, Beveridge J **Flexor tendon injuries of the hand** Curr Orthop 1986;1:91–99

Ejeskar A, **Flexor tendon repair in no-man's-land: results of primary repair with controlled mobilisation** J Hand Surg [Am] 1984;9-A:171–177

Operative Technique

Richards HJ **Primary repair of the divided digital flexor tendon** In: Birch R, Brooks D, ed. The hand. 4th edn (Rob and Smith's Operative Surgery) London: Butterworth, 1984:121–129

Varian JPW **Tendon injuries in the hand** In: Birch R, Brooks D, ed. The hand. 4th edn (Rob and Smith's Operative Surgery) London: Butterworth, 1984:130–148

Tendon Grafting

Boyes JH, Stark HH **Flexor-tendon grafts in the fingers and thumb. A study of factors influencing results in 1000 cases** J Bone Joint Surg [Am] 1971; 53-A:1332–1342

Review Article

Lamb DW **Injuries of the flexor tendons** In: Lamb DW, Hooper G, Kuczynski K, ed. The practice of hand surgery. 2nd edn Oxford: Blackwell Scientific Publications, 1989; 172–184

Kleinert gave a short review of the subject with a description of operative technique within the flexor digital sheath. The repaired tendon is protected with a dynamic splint constructed at the end of the operation. In repairs in "no-man's-land", **Lister** later reported 75% good or excellent results. These studies have been recently updated by **Tubiana** who included discussion on flexor tendon grafting and injuries to the flexor pollicis longus. **Ejeskar** showed that repair of isolated profundus lesions could be done primarily or secondarily within one month of injury with equally good results. The results of reconstruction of flexor tendons in the fingers are unpredictable. Failure is common and usually a consequence of adhesions between the tendon and the sheath.

Most older orthopaedic surgeons have been brought up on the use of tendon grafts and **Boyes'** study described the factors which influence the results. Scarring from injury or failed primary reparative procedures compromised the results of secondary tendon grafting. Palmaris longus was the best donor tendon. Although excellent results are obtained with tendon grafting by those with special expertise (**Pulvertaft** and **Boyes**), the results of tendon grafting are often poor. There is now a trend towards primary flexor-tendon suture and this is described by **Richards** and **Varian**.

In a recent review article, **Lamb** has discussed both the technique and results of the alternative methods of management. Tenolysis and recent advances with the use of artificial tendons were also reviewed.

Extensor Tendon Injuries

Mallet Finger

Stack HG **Mallet finger** Hand 1969;1:83–89

Moss JG, Steingold RF **The long-term result of mallet finger injury. A retrospective study of 100 cases** Hand 1983;15:151–154

Stark HH, Gainor BJ, Ashworth CR, Zemel NP, Rickard TA **Operative treatment of intra-articular fractures of the dorsal aspect of the distal phalanx of the digits** J Bone Joint Surg [Am] 1987;69-A:892–896

Burke FD **Editorial: Mallet finger** J Hand Surg [Br] 1988;13-B:115–117

The paper by **Stack** described the anatomy and pathology of this injury. Conservative treatment with a simple polythene splint is described and some indications for operative treatment discussed. The paper by **Moss** reviewed 100 patients three years after injury; 29 patients still had symptoms, consisting mainly of pain and cold intolerance. The degree of residual deformity, presence of a fracture or delay in treatment were not related to symptoms. **Stark** described fractures of the distal phalanx involving more than one-third of the dorsal articular surface, treated by open reduction and K-wire fixation and reported that exact reduction and internal fixation resulted in excellent function. The management of mallet finger deformity continues to provoke discussion in journals and conferences and the debate is summarised in a recent editorial by **Burke**.

The Boutonnière Deformity

Matev I **The boutonnière deformity** Hand 1969;1:90–95

Souter WA **The problem of boutonnière deformity** Clin Orthop 1974;104:116–133

Rupture of the Extensor Pollicis Longus Tendon

Helal B, Chen SC, Iwegbu G **Rupture of the extensor pollicis longus tendon in undisplaced Colles' type of fracture** Hand 1982;14:41–47

Operative Technique

Varian JPW **Tendon injuries in the hand** In: Birch R, Brooks D, ed. The Hand. 4th edn (Rob and Smith's Operative Surgery) London: Butterworth, 1984:130–148

Review Article

Hooper G **Injuries of the extensor tendons** In: Lamb DW, Hooper G, Kuczynski K, ed. The practice of hand surgery. 2nd edn Oxford: Blackwell Scientific Publications, 1989: 184–195

Matev described the anatomy and pathodynamics of the boutonnière deformity. Conservative treatment was effective in early cases when initiated up to three weeks after injury. Possible reconstructive operations for the difficult late case are discussed. **Souter** presented a comprehensive review of this subject and advocated a conservative approach for those presenting early, but operative treatment for those presenting after three months.

Helal showed that there is a higher risk that the tendon of extensor pollicis longus will rupture after an undisplaced Colles' fracture compared with those which are displaced. The transfer of the extensor indicis proprius tendon gave consistently excellent results. **Varian**'s chapter illustrated the techniques for extensor repair at various sites on the dorsum of the hand. **Hooper** has summarised the treatment of injuries of the extensor tendons at different levels. The controversial methods of reconstruction of late mallet and late boutonnière deformity are discussed.

Nerve Injuries in the Hand

Milford L **Nerve injuries** In: Crenshaw AH, ed. Campbell's operative orthopaedics. 7th edn, Vol. 1 St. Louis: CV Mosby, 1987:229–239

Honner R, Fragiadakis EG, Lamb DW **An investigation of the factors affecting the results of digital nerve division** Hand 1970;2:21–30

Millesi H, Meissl G, Berger A **The interfascicular nerve grafting of the median and ulnar nerves** J Bone Joint Surg [Am] 1972;54-A:727–750

Poppen NK, McCarroll HR, Doyle JR, Niebauer JJ **Recovery of sensibility after suture of digital nerves** J Hand Surg 1979;4:212–225

Wynn Parry CB, Harper D, Fletcher I, Dean AE, Knight PN, Robinson AR **New types of lively splints for peripheral nerve lesions affecting the hand** Hand 1970;2:31–38

Milford has provided a comprehensive review of the assessment and treatment of peripheral nerve injuries in the hand and wrist. The indications for primary nerve suture and secondary nerve repair are considered as well as the value of neurovascular island grafts.

Honner reviewed the results of complete nerve division in 51 patients treated by primary or by secondary suture. The best results were obtained in skilled workers with a primary repair. There were only four good results out of 32 with a secondary repair. The results became more unsatisfactory as the site of injury proceeded distally.

Millesi discussed the operative technique of nerve grafting and reviewed the results of 202 nerve grafts for median and ulnar nerve division. He concluded that nerve grafting without tension gave better results than end-to-end suture under tension and that microscopic repair is required.

Recovery of sensibility after epineurial suture of 74 digital nerves was studied by **Poppen**. Two point discrimination was found to be the best method of testing sensibility recovery. The patient's age at the time of nerve suture was directly related to the return of sensibility.

Wynn Parry has described splints for a drop wrist, claw hand, intrinsic and thenar paralysis. Principles concerning nerve injuries and also those of rehabilitation are considered in the appropriate sections elsewhere (pp 20–22,65).

Finger Tip Injuries and Amputations

Clinical Studies

Milford L **Amputations** In: Crenshaw AH, ed. Campbell's operative orthopaedics. 7th edn, Vol. 1 St. Louis: CV Mosby, 1987:291–305

Scott JE **Amputation of the finger** Br J Surg 1974;61:574–576

Murray JF **Amputations** In: McFarlane RM, ed. Unsatisfactory results in hand surgery Edinburgh, etc: Churchill Livingstone, 1987:141–157

Das SK, Brown HG **The management of lost finger tips in children** Hand 1978;10:16–27

Carroll RE **Ring injuries in the hand** Clin Orthop 1974;104:175–182

Amputations of the Thumb

Campbell Reid DA **Thumb injuries** Hand 1970;2:126–129

Pringle RG **Amputations of the thumb: a study of techniques of repair and residual disability** Injury 1972;3:211–217

Ratliff AHC **Amputations of the distal part of the thumb** Hand 1972;4:190–193

Morrison WA, O'Brien BM, MacLeod AM **Experience with thumb reconstruction** J Hand Surg [Br] 1984;9-B:223–233

Operative Technique

Burke FD **Finger tip injuries and amputations** In: Birch R, Brooks DM, ed. The Hand. 4th edn (Rob and Smith's Operative Surgery) London: Butterworth, 1984:210–225

Milford has provided a general chapter on the principles of amputation of fingers and discussed the various techniques available for amputations of the fingertip including re-amputation, free skin graft, the Kutler flap and thenar flaps. Amputations of multiple digits are also carefully considered. The latter part of this chapter concerned with reconstructions after amputation has not been considered since this is the province of the very specialised hand surgeon. **Scott** stressed the importance of obtaining a non-tender cover of the stump and that length should be sacrificed to obtain this. **Murray** emphasised that there were a significant number of poor results and that complications of finger amputations are distressing and commonplace. The special problem of amputation of the tips of fingers in children was studied by **Das** who analysed 60 injuries. The conservative method of treatment is considered to be the best. The finger was left to heal with regular dressings. A ring on the finger may cause a severe injury when caught by a projecting object. **Carroll** has described four types of injury which may result with the appropriate management.

Amputations of the thumb are classified according to the level of thumb loss by **Campbell Reid**. Where amputation is distal to the metacarpophalangeal joint with an adequate length of thumb, primary skin cover is recommended and minimal shortening only permissible. **Pringle** performed a retrospective study of 20 patients who had suffered partial amputation of the thumb and noted that the residual disability is generally slight. **Ratliff** noted that where a mobile non-sensitive stump was achieved, disability after an amputation of the terminal part of the thumb was often minor. The surgical treatment of major thumb loss is not usually considered the realm of the orthopaedic surgeon. Nevertheless, the paper by **Morrison** has been included since unique experience is recorded on this important and difficult subject.

Details of operative technique for fingertip injuries and amputations including assessment and anaethesia are described by **Burke**.

High Pressure Injection Injuries

Kaufman HD **High pressure injection injuries** In: Birch R, Brooks D, ed. The hand. 4th edn (Rob and Smith's Operative Surgery) London: Butterworth, 1984: 85–91

Injection of foreign material – loosely called "grease gun injuries" – into the tissues under high pressure is rare. Even with immediate skilled treatment, permanent severe damage may result. **Kaufman** has provided a useful reference based on a study of 51 cases.

Infections in the Hand

Clinical Studies

Burke FD **Infection of the hand** Curr Orthop 1987;1:209–218

Leddy JE **Review article: infections of the upper extremity** J Hand Surg [Am] 1986;11-A:294–297

Glass KD **Factors related to the resolution of treated hand infections** J Hand Surg [Am] 1982;7-A:388–394

Specific Problems

Pollen AG **Acute infection of the tendon sheaths** Hand 1974;6:21–25

Rashkoff ES, Burkhalter WE, Mann RJ **Septic arthritis of the wrist** J Bone Joint Surg [Am] 1983;65-A:824–828

Chuinard RG, D'Ambrosia RD **Human bite infections of the hand** J Bone Joint Surg [Am] 1977;59-A:416–418

Dreyfuss UY, Singer M **Human bites of the hand. A study of 106 patients**
J Hand Surg [Am] 1985;10-A:884–889

Operative Technique

Sneddon J **Infections** In: Birch R, Brooks DM, ed. The hand. 4th edn (Rob and
Smith's Operative Surgery) London: Butterworth, 1984:108–120

Adams JC **Drainage incisions for acute suppurating infections of the fascial
spaces of the hand** In: Standard orthopaedic operations, 3rd edn Edinburgh, etc:
Churchill Livingstone, 1985:239–243

Burke's review article covered the principles and specific management of hand
wounds and infections. The paper by **Leddy** outlined the bacteriology and antibiotic
therapy required for each infection. Despite effective antibiotics, infections continue
to be a serious problem. Relatively rare lesions such as an haematogenous septic
arthritis, infections in drug addicts and those due to gram negative organisms are also
included. **Glass** noted the resolution time of infection of the hand was slow, 8 days or
longer in 57% of 135 patients. Factors affecting the speed of resolution included delay
in treatment, adequacy of surgical drainage and efficacy of antibiotics.

Infections of tendon sheaths have been specifically mentioned in **Pollen**'s article in
view of the appreciation of the value of early diagnosis and surgical treatment. The rare
problem of septic arthritis is discussed by **Rashkoff**. He recommended that the wrist
should be aspirated early and that with appropriate intravenous antibiotics and surgical
drainage, a good result can be achieved. Bite infections of the hand appear to have
become an increasing problem. **Chuinard** studied 59 cases caused by human bites.
There is a high potential for serious complications and cephalosporins are advocated
as the correct antibiotic therapy. **Dreyfuss** considered that the most important factor
governing the final result of treatment was the time interval between injury and
commencement of treatment; the morbidity rate of these injuries was considerable.

Sneddon's chapter gives a comprehensive, well illustrated review of surgical
procedures necessary to treat hand infections and this chapter is complemented by that
written by **Adams** which also illustrates the anatomical spaces in the hand.

Replantation

Godfrey AM, Lister GD, Kleinert HE **Replantation of the digits and hand**
In: Birch R, Brooks DM, ed. The Hand. 4th edn (Rob and Smith's Operative
Surgery) London: Butterworth, 1984:71–81

Replantation demands highly specialised training and appropriate facilities. It is not intended to study this subject in detail in this book, but to provide a rapid source of knowledge. **Godfrey** has described in detail the pre-operative and operative technique for replantation of the digits and the hand and briefly summarised the results in an experience of 200 cases between 1975 and 1980.

Rehabilitation

Wynn Parry CB **Rehabilitation of the hand**. 4th edn London: Butterworth, 1981

In an impressive textbook which has gone to four editions, **Wynn Parry** discussed all aspects of rehabilitation of the hand. We would particularly draw attention to the sections on re-education after peripheral nerve injuries, causalgia, management of the stiff hand and those on physiotherapy and occupational therapy.

Section 4
The Spine

THE SPINE

Classification and Mechanisms of Injury

Holdsworth Sir F **Fractures, dislocations and fracture-dislocations of the spine** J Bone Joint Surg [Am] 1970;52-A:1534–1551

Denis F **Spinal instability as defined by the three-column spine concept in acute spinal trauma** Clin Orthop 1984;189:65–76

Holdsworth, in a classical paper, summarised a study of injuries of the spine based on observations of over 1000 patients. A classification of these injuries was presented and illustrated and he emphasised that precise diagnosis, both bony and neurological, was fundamental. For assessment of prognosis in thoracolumbar injuries, it was important to distinguish between cord and root damage. Holdsworth divided these injuries into two groups, stable and unstable and considered they were injuries of two columns – anterior (vertebral body) and posterior (the facet joints and posterior ligament complex).

   Denis has developed the concept of a three column spine based on a study of 412 injuries of the thoracolumbar spine. Holdsworth's classification is amplified to include a middle column consisting of the posterior longitudinal ligament, the posterior annulus fibrosis and the posterior wall of the vertebral body. Spinal fractures are classified into four different categories: compression, burst, seat belt and fracture dislocations.

Spinal Cord Injury

Silver JR **Immediate management of spinal injuries** Br J Hosp Med 1983;29:412–425

Grundy D, Russell J, Swain A **ABC of spinal cord injury** London: British Medical Journal Publications, 1986

Bedbrook GM **Spinal injuries with tetraplegia and paraplegia** J Bone Joint Surg [Br] 1979;61-B:267–284

Silver described a regimen for immediate management of spinal injury based on experience of 421 patients treated at the National Spinal Injuries Centre at Stoke Mandeville from 1970 to 1983. A short, clear description is provided, discussing the transport and position of the patient, the early treatment including that of associated injuries and briefly, the outcome.

Grundy and his colleagues in 1986 edited the ABC of Spinal Cord Injury, a small book of 56 pages in which a number of articles previously published in the British Medical Journal have been collected. Fourteen extensively illustrated sections contain didactic instruction on the practical investigation, early and late management of the paraplegic patient.

Bedbrook, in a review article, marshalled his experience of spinal injuries and discussed the controversy over conservative and surgical management of acute thoracolumbar injuries with paraplegia. This paper has also been included because of the bibliography which gives references to the well known contributions of Guttmann.

Injuries of the Cervical Spine

Clinical Studies and Pathology (C3 – C7)

Bohlman HH Acute fractures and dislocations of the cervical spine: an analysis of 300 hospitalised patients and review of the literature J Bone Joint Surg [Am] 1979;61-A:1119–1142

Harris JH, Edeiken-Monroe B, Kopaniky DR A practical classification of acute cervical spine injuries Orthop Clin North Am 1986;17:15–30

Stauffer ES Diagnosis and prognosis of acute cervical spinal cord injury Clin Orthop 1975;112:9–15

Marar BC The pattern of neurological damage as an aid to the diagnosis of the mechanism in cervical spine injuries J Bone Joint Surg [Am] 1974; 56-A:1648–1654

Bohlman stressed the dangers of a laminectomy and concluded that reduction and fusion offered the best chance for recovery of neural function and restoration of stability. A comprehensive classification of cervical spine injuries based on the mechanism of injury is presented by **Harris**. **Stauffer** discussed the early diagnosis and type and severity of spinal cord damage with brief reference to the accurate initial examination and the significance of return of involuntary reflex activity. **Marar** studied 126 cases of cervical spine injuries and described five groups according to the clinical pattern of neurological damage, referring particularly to the anterior spinal cord injury previously described by Schneider. The patterns were related to the bone injury and the prognosis of the spinal cord deficiency correlated with the mechanism of injury.

Treatment (C3 – C7)

Grundy DJ **Skull traction and its complications** Injury 1983;15:173–177

Evans DK **Reduction of cervical dislocations** J Bone Joint Surg [Br] 1961; 43-B:552–555

Kostuik JP **Indications for the use of the halo immobilisation** Clin Orthop 1981;154:46–50

Burke DC, Berryman D **The place of closed manipulation in the management of flexion-rotation dislocations of the cervical spine** J Bone Joint Surg [Br] 1971; 53-B:165–182

Hamblen DL **Anterior fusion of the cervical spine** In: Bentley G, ed. Orthopaedics. Part 1, 3rd edn. (Rob and Smith's Operative Surgery) London: Butterworth, 1979:347–354

Hamblen DL **Posterior fusions of the cervical spine** In: Bentley G, ed. Orthopaedics. Part 1, 3rd edn. (Rob and Smith's Operative Surgery) London: Butterworth, 1979:355–365

Stauffer ES, Kelly EG **Fracture-dislocation of the cervical spine – instability and recurrent deformity following treatment by anterior inter-body fusion** J Bone Joint Surg [Am] 1977;59-A:45–48

Johnson RM, Owen JR, Dennis BA, Hart L, Callahan RA **Cervical orthoses: a guide to their selection and use** Clin Orthop 1981;154:34–45

Evans DK **Dislocations at the cervicothoracic junction** J Bone Joint Surg [Br] 1983;65-B:124–127

Grundy described the use of skull traction and its complications in 391 patients over a seven-year period in a spinal injuries unit. Although thought to be a minor procedure, complications occurred in 37% of patients. The complication rate was lowest using the Cone Caliper. **Evans** discussed the use of manual reduction under general anaesthesia of 17 patients with cervical dislocations. Emphasis was placed on the disadvantages of slow reduction by traction. The method of halo immobilisation with its indications, technique and complications is briefly described by **Kostuik**.

Manipulative treatment was described by **Burke** in 76 dislocations of the cervical spine. The reduction was maintained by skeletal traction. The low incidence of late instability after conservative treatment was stressed and the place of surgery in the management of these injuries outlined. The practical details of operative approach and possible techniques for anterior and posterior fusion are illustrated by **Hamblen**. Recurrence of angular deformity with instability was described by **Stauffer** in a retrospective study of 16 patients. Anterior fusion should not be performed where there is evidence of disruption of posterior ligaments. **Johnson** illustrated the various types of orthosis that may be used. **Evans** considered that dislocations at the cervicothoracic junction may frequently be missed. When diagnosed, open reduction is necessary.

Hyperextension Injuries

Burke DC **Hyperextension injuries of the spine** J Bone Joint Surg [Br] 1971; 53-B:3–12

Marar BC **Hyperextension injuries of the cervical spine: the pathogenesis of damage to the spinal cord** J Bone Joint Surg [Am] 1974;56-A:1655–1662

Norris SH, Watt I **The prognosis of neck injuries resulting from rear-end vehicle collisions** J Bone Joint Surg [Br] 1983;65-B:608–611

Burke studied a series of 51 extension injuries of the cervical spine and four with extension injuries at the thoracolumbar junction and discussed the different patterns of hyperextension injury, based on the pathological anatomy. **Marar** discussed the pathogenesis of cord damage in 45 patients with a hyperextension injury of the cervical spine including four who died with this injury. He considered the mechanism of injury was a combination of hyperextension and backward shearing. The paper by **Norris** discussed the prolonged disability and litigation which may follow these injuries. He divided the so-called "whiplash injuries" into three groups and considered that in the worst group, where there was a reduction of cervical movement and objective neurological loss, only 10% of these patients were entirely free of symptoms two years after injury.

Fractures of the Odontoid

Anderson LD, D'Alonzo RT **Fractures of the odontoid process of the axis** J Bone Joint Surg [Am] 1974;56-A:1663–1674

Clark CR, White AA **Fractures of the dens: A multi-centre study** J Bone Joint Surg [Am] 1985;67-A:1340–1348

McGraw RW, Rusch RM **Atlanto-axial arthrodesis** J Bone Joint Surg [Br] 1973;55-B:482–489

Anderson studied a series of 49 fractures and classified these into three types. Fractures of the body were prone to non-union and surgery in the form of spinal fusion was commonly required in this group. **Clark** noted that treatment of these fractures was often inadequate and management was controversial. He agreed with the classification described by Anderson but observed that initial management of the type II fractures with a halo device was successful in only 68%. Posterior cervical fusion was successful in 96% and was therefore considered to be the treatment of choice. **McGraw** defined the indications for atlanto-axial arthrodesis and described in detail a precise technique for the performance of this operation.

Hangman's Fracture

Effendi B, Roy D, Cornish B, Dussault RG, Laurin CA **Fractures of the ring of the axis: a classification based on the analysis of 131 cases** J Bone Joint Surg [Br] 1981;63-B:319–327

A retrospective analysis of 131 patients suffering from a fracture of the ring of the axis is reported. The injury was classified into three types according to the radiological displacement and stability. Guidelines for the management of these difficult injuries were discussed and well illustrated. A fracture of the ring of the axis is usually benign but, nonetheless, a mortality of 7% is reported.

Cervical Instability

Herkowitz HN, Rothman RH **Subacute instability of the cervical spine** Spine 1984;9:348–357

White AA, Panjabi MM **The role of stabilization in the treatment of cervical spine injuries** Spine 1984;9:512–522

Webb JK, Broughton RBK, McSweeney T, Park WM **Hidden flexion injury of the cervical spine** J Bone Joint Surg [Br] 1976;58-B:322–327

Evans DK **Anterior cervical subluxation** J Bone Joint Surg [Br] 1976; 58-B:318–321

Four papers have been included which demonstrate increased interest in cervical instability. **Herkowitz** described six patients where initial radiographs showed no bony or soft tissue abnormality. **White** discussed the various types of stabilisation which could be performed including anterior and posterior fusion. **Webb** described seven patients who developed unexpected late vertebral deformity after flexion injuries. Four radiological signs were noted that suggested posterior cervical complex damage. They included widening of the interspinous space, mild intervertebral subluxation and loss of the normal cervical lordosis. In an adjacent paper, **Evans** also noted that anterior subluxation of the cervical spine from flexion rotational violence is often overlooked. Four patients required stabilisation by operation, in contrast with complete dislocations where 80%–90% fuse spontaneously.

Cervical Spine Injuries in Children

Cattell HS, Filtzer DL **Pseudosubluxation and other normal variations in the cervical spine in children – a study of 160 children** J Bone Joint Surg [Am] 1965;47-A:1295–1309

Fielding JW, Hawkins RJ **Atlanto-axial rotatory fixation (fixed rotatory subluxation of the atlanto-axial joint)** J Bone Surg [Am] 1977;59-A:37–44

Sherk HH, Nicholson JT, Chung SMK **Fractures of the odontoid process in young children** J Bone Joint Surg [Am] 1978;60-A:921–924

In the diagnosis of neck injuries in children there are several well known radiological pitfalls. **Cattell** has considered this subject by studying the cervical spines of 160 normal children. Possible normal variations were observed which might otherwise have been regarded as pathological. Irreducible subluxation at the atlanto-axial joint is described by **Fielding** in 17 cases. All patients had a torticollis and restricted, painful neck motion. Treatment included skull traction followed by atlanto-axial arthrodesis if necessary. **Sherk** has drawn attention to the problems presented by fractures of the odontoid process in children. These fractures almost always heal with support in a Minerva jacket or halo cast.

The Paralysed Upper Limb

Lamb DW, Chan KM **Surgical reconstruction of the upper limb in traumatic tetraplegia: a review of 41 patients** J Bone Joint Surg [Br] 1983;65-B:291–298

Lamb presented a review of 41 patients with traumatic tetraplegia on whom reconstructive surgery of the upper limb was carried out. Twelve patients were followed for more than 10 years and a detailed discussion is provided of the value of surgery in these difficult cases.

Injuries of the Thoracolumbar Spine

Radiology

Keene JS, Goletz TH, Lilleas F, Alter AJ, Sackett JF **Diagnosis of vertebral fractures: a comparison of conventional radiography, conventional tomography and computed axial tomography** J Bone Joint Surg [Am] 1982; 64-A:586–595

McAfee PC, Yuan HA, Fredrickson BE, Lubicky JP **The value of computed tomography in thoracolumbar fractures: an analysis of 100 consecutive cases and a new classification** J Bone Joint Surg [Am] 1983;65-A:461–473

Considerable attention has recently been focused on the accurate diagnosis of fractures at the thoracolumbar level of the spine and this is reflected in the papers by both **Keene** and **McAfee**. Computerized axial scans provide a better display of the neural canal without change of the position of the patient and therefore with less risk. **McAfee** studied 100 consecutive patients with potentially unstable fractures, analysed degrees of instability and particularly middle column failure in unstable burst fractures.

Treatment

Nicoll EA **Fractures of the dorso-lumbar spine** J Bone Joint Surg [Br] 1949; 31-B:376–394

Bedbrook GM **Treatment of thoracolumbar dislocation and fractures with paraplegia** Clin Orthop 1975:112:27–43

Lewis J, McKibbin B **The treatment of unstable fracture dislocations of the thoracolumbar spine accompanied by paraplegia** J Bone Joint Surg [Br] 1974; 56-B:603–612

Bohlman HH **Current concepts review: treatment of fractures and dislocations of the thoracic and lumbar spine** J Bone Joint Surg [Am] 1985;67-A:165–169

Stauffer ES **Current concepts review: internal fixation of fractures of the thoracolumbar spine** J Bone Joint Surg [Am] 1984;66-A:1136–1138

Gertzbein SD, MacMichael D, Tile M **Harrington instrumentation as a method of fixation in fractures of the spine: a critical analysis of deficiencies** J Bone Joint Surg [Br] 1982;64-B:526–529

McAfee PC, Bohlman HH **Complications following Harrington instrumentation for fractures of the thoracolumbar spine** J Bone Joint Surg [Am] 1985;67-A:672–686

Gaines RW, Breedlove RF, Munson G **Stabilization of thoracic and thoracolumbar fracture-dislocations with Harrington rods and sub-laminar wires** Clin Orthop 1984;189:195–203

McAfee PC, Bohlman HH, Yuan HA **Anterior decompression of traumatic thoracolumbar fractures with incomplete neurological deficit using a retroperitoneal approach** J Bone Joint Surg [Am] 1985;67-A:89–104

Kostuik JP **Anterior fixation for fractures of the thoracic and lumbar spine with or without neurologic involvement** Clin Orthop 1984;189:103–115

Riska EB, Myllynen P, Bostman O **Antero-lateral decompression for neural involvement in thoracolumbar fractures – a review of 78 cases** J Bone Joint Surg [Br] 1987;69-B:704–708

Nicoll studied the results of conservative treatment of 166 fractures in miners. Disability was analysed in terms of pain, mobility, power and endurance. **Bedbrook** in 1975 described with illustrations the practical conservative management of paraplegia due to injuries at this level. He stated that 90% of fractures of the dorsal lumbar spine with paraparesis or paraplegia can best be reduced by closed methods when satisfactory alignment can be obtained. 'The use of spinal rods and clamps is rarely indicated'.

There has been a remarkable change in approach to the management of these injuries in the past two decades. **Lewis** marshalled the arguments for and against surgery and then compared the results of treatment in two unselected series of patients with unstable fractures. One group had been treated by conservative methods, the other subjected to open reduction and internal fixation with double plates. No difference in the amount of neurological recovery could be detected but in those treated by plating, there was no pain and improved function. **Bohlman** advocated the use of internal fixation for unstable fractures whether or not a neurological defect was present.

Stauffer discussed the various types of posterior instrumentation including that of Harrington and Luque. The value of decompression and the controversial subject of length of fusion is debated. **Gertzbein** studied the results of use of Harrington rods in both double distraction and double compression. With burst fractures where the anterior pillar was deficient, there was a significant loss of reduction. **McAfee** illustrated significant complications in 40 patients; the series was a collected one and 35 of the operations had been performed elsewhere. The reader is left in no doubt of the difficulties of Harrington instrumentation.

Gaines described the management of 17 unstable injuries with Harrington double distraction rod technique supplemented by double 18 gauge wires applied to two intact laminae above and below the injury. This paper gives a precise description of the indications for this operation and also a summary of the operative technique.

McAfee, in another paper, discussed the results of anterior decompression of thoracolumbar fractures with an incomplete neurological deficit. Forty-eight patients were followed for an average of three years. Post-operative decompression was proved by diagnostic computed tomography. The degree of neurological recovery was impressive.

Kostuik discussed the trend towards the anterior approach for early and late thoracic and lumbar spine burst fractures with a description of the results of treatment on 49 patients.

Neurological recovery following antero-lateral decompression was analysed by

Riska in 78 patients. The best results were in burst fractures when a detached fragment of a vertebral body had been displaced into the spinal canal.

Fractures of the Pelvis

The Classic

Holdsworth FW **Dislocation and fracture-dislocation of the pelvis** J Bone Joint Surg [Br] 1948;30-B:461–466

Pathological Anatomy

Bucholz RW **The pathological anatomy of Malgaigne fracture-dislocation of the pelvis** J Bone Joint Surg [Am] 1981;63-A:400–404

Holdsworth reviewed 50 dislocations and fracture-dislocations of the pelvis. One-half of the 27 patients with a sacro-iliac dislocation had significant pain and were unable to return to heavy work. The prognosis in fracture dislocation was good and nearly all patients went back to heavy work. Conservative treatment with longitudinal traction and pelvic slings was illustrated.

Bucholz studied the pathological anatomy in 32 patients who had died with these injuries. Posterior lesions at autopsy were found in all patients with pelvic trauma even when the radiographs had revealed only an anterior lesion.

Clinical Studies

Monahan PRW, Taylor RG **Dislocation and fracture-dislocation of the pelvis** Injury 1975;6:325–333

Pennal GF, Massiah KA **Non-union and delayed union of fractures of the pelvis** Clin Orthop 1980;151:124–129

McMurtry R, Saibil E **General assessment and management of the polytraumatised patient.** In: Tile M, ed. Fractures of the pelvis and acetabulum Baltimore: Williams and Wilkins, 1984:41–55

Tile M **External fixation** In: Fractures of the pelvis and acetabulum Baltimore: Williams and Wilkins, 1984:121–131

Goldstein A, Phillips T, Sclafani SJA, Scalea T, Duncan A, Goldstein J, Panetta T, Shaftan G **Early open reduction and internal fixation of the disrupted pelvic ring** J Trauma 1986;26:325–333

Tile M **Pelvic ring fractures. Should they be fixed?** J Bone Joint Surg [Br] 1988;70-B:1–12

The natural history of these major injuries has been stressed by **Tile** in his 1988 article based on a review of 248 cases. Stable injuries gave few major long-term problems. By contrast, patients with vertical unstable pelvic disruptions had many problems including continuing pain especially posteriorly, mal-union and non-union. The results of a series of 43 patients all treated conservatively were described by **Monahan**. One-half had associated skeletal injuries and 44% had barely recordable or unrecordable blood pressure on admission. Persistent posterior lumbosacral or sacro-iliac pain was stressed. **Pennal** drew attention to non-union and delayed union as a cause for persistent symptoms in a series of 42 patients.

McMurtry described the general assessment and treatment based on simultaneous care and a protocol outlined by the topical Advanced Trauma Life Support Programme of the American College of Surgeons. The increased use of external fixation is discussed by **Tile** in his book. Although an unstable pelvic ring disruption cannot be fully stabilised by an anterior frame, these patients are often very ill and a simple frame configuration is preferred. The use of early open reduction and internal fixation is described by **Goldstein** in 33 patients. An aggressive approach is advocated but the surgery is complicated and has to be learned with special training. It is considered to be safe and offers advantages in the acute management of multiply injured patients with a decreased incidence of respiratory failure.

Tile in a 1988 review article debated the pros and cons for fixation of pelvic ring fractures. The indications for both external fixation and open reduction and internal fixation for the various types of pelvic injury are summarised. He concluded that in a series of 494 pelvic fractures treated over a five-year period, only 19% needed stabilisation, and this was by internal fixation in only 5%. When open reduction is required an anterior approach to the sacro-iliac joint is favoured.

Bladder and Urethra

Mitchell JP **Trauma to the urethra** Injury 1975;7:84–88

Mitchell JP **Urinary tract trauma** Bristol: J Wright, 1984:144–155 (management of suspected bladder rupture), 178–205 (diagnosis of rupture of the posterior urethra and surgical management of rupture of the posterior urethra)

The management of damage to the urethra is discussed by **Mitchell** (in *Injury*). The passage of a catheter is condemned as clinically misleading. Partial rupture is considered to be relatively common and thus primary treatment recommended is usually suprapubic diversion. Mitchell has recently published an authoritative monograph on injuries of the urinary tract based on his unique experience. The book provides much useful practical information concerning the diagnosis and management of these injuries.

Section 5
The Lower Limb

Dislocations of the Hip and Fractures of the Acetabulum

The Classic

Epstein HC **Traumatic dislocations of the hip** Clin Orthop 1973;92:116–142

Long-Term Results

Rowe CR, Lowell JD **Prognosis of fractures of the acetabulum** J Bone Joint Surg [Am] 1961;43-A:30–59

Epstein HC **Posterior fracture-dislocations of the hip – long-term follow-up** J Bone Joint Surg [Am] 1974;56-A:1103–1127

Upadhyay SS, Moulton A **The long-term results of traumatic posterior dislocation of the hip** J Bone Joint Surg [Br] 1981;63-B:548–551

The papers by **Epstein** are classics. The first describes the natural history with complications of 426 cases including 42 children. With the more complicated fracture-dislocation primary open reduction appeared to give better results, with reduced incidence of complications such as avascular necrosis or traumatic arthritis. The second paper presents the results of treatment of 150 cases followed for an average of 7 years.

Rowe in 1961 published an end-result study of 93 fractures of the acetabulum observed for an average of six years. The prognosis was more favourable than previously expected. The outcome depended primarily on the condition of the dome or weight-bearing portion of the acetabulum. The clinical and radiological findings at one year after injury were a reliable guide to the ultimate prognosis of the hip. The work by **Upadhyay** is included since it gives the important message that 25% of simple posterior dislocations have a poor long-term result.

Management

Tipton WW, D'Ambrosia RD, Ryle DP **Non-operative management of central fracture dislocations of the hip** J Bone Joint Surg [Am] 1975;57-A:888–893

Letournel E **Acetabulum fractures – classification and management** Clin Orthop 1980;151:81–106

Tile M **Fractures of the pelvis and acetabulum** Baltimore: Williams and Wilkins, 1984:177–247 Chap 15 (classification), Chap 16 (assessment and surgical indications), Chap 17 (management)

Matta JM, Lowell M, Anderson MD, Epstein HC, Hendricks P **Fractures of the acetabulum – a retrospective analysis** Clin Orthop 1986;205:230–240

Canale ST, Manugian AH **Irreducible traumatic dislocations of the hip** J Bone Joint Surg [Am] 1979;61-A:7–14

Lang-Stevenson A, Getty CJM **The Pipkin fracture-dislocation of the hip** Injury 1987;18:264–269

Review Article

Tile M **Fractures of the acetabulum** In: Schatzker J, Tile M, ed. The rationale of operative fracture care Berlin, etc: Springer-Verlag, 1987:173–213

There is controversy over the subject of conservative treatment versus operation in the management of central fracture dislocation of the hip joint. **Tipton** carried out a follow-up study of 24 patients and discussed the use of skeletal traction on the femur to maintain reduction. With a completely different and essentially operative approach, **Letournel** discussed experience with a new classification of fractures of the acetabulum, essentially defining injuries of the anterior column, the posterior column and complex transverse fractures. From 1955 to 1978, 582 acetabular fractures were operated upon and technique, complications and results presented. A perfect open reduction is considered to be the method of choice to treat displaced acetabular fractures. **Tile** amplified this classification and in a lucid chapter (Chapter 15) illustrated each type with a diagram, radiographs and CT scan. Assessment, surgical indications and management are then discussed in subsequent chapters (Chaps. 16 and 17).

Matta has recently reported results of a study of 204 acetabular fractures, evaluated both clinically and radiologically with a follow-up of approximately four years. The radiological result usually correlated with a clinical result. Stress is given not only to the reduction of the fracture and its maintenance, but also its relation with the weight-bearing dome of the acetabulum. A good result can be expected providing both these features are achieved either by operation or by conservative treatment. Matta concluded that open reduction and internal fixation may be recommended for many displaced acetabular fractures but that this requires surgeons with special interest and training.

Canale reviewed the results of treatment of 54 dislocations and noted that nine required open reduction, after either a failed attempt at closed reduction or one that was not concentric. The importance of a stable concentric reduction is emphasised.

The various types of fracture of the head of the femur which may occur in association with a dislocation were described by Pipkin in 1957. The injury is rare and treatment controversial. **Lang-Stevenson** reviewed seven cases, illustrated the Pipkin classification and advocated surgical treatment.

Tile has recently published an excellent chapter on fractures of the acetabulum (1987) which provides a recent update on this subject. The authors of this book would particularly like to draw attention to the description of the various surgical approaches which are clearly illustrated (pp. 200–213).

Hip Fractures in the Elderly

Historical

Cooper A **A treatise on dislocations and on fractures of the joints.** 4th edn London: Longman, Hurst, Rhys, Orme and Browne, 1824: plate XIII

Basic Science

Crock HV **An atlas of the arterial supply of the head and neck of the femur in man** Clin Orthop 1980;152:17–27

Catto M **A histological study of avascular necrosis of the femoral head after transcervical fracture** J Bone Joint Surg [Br] 1965;47-B:749–776

Catto M **The histological appearances of late segmental collapse of the femoral head after transcervical fracture** J Bone Joint Surg [Br] 1965; 47-B:777–791

The characteristics of a fracture of the femoral neck were demonstrated more than 150 years ago by **Astley Cooper** (1824). Recognition of the injury inflicted on the vascular supply to the femoral head by an intracapsular fracture led Cooper to the conclusion that this fracture would not unite. The precise blood supply has been beautifully illustrated by **Crock. Catto** examined the femoral heads of 109 patients removed more than 16 days after fracture. She noted that some femoral heads became completely necrotic whilst others were only partly affected. Necrotic bone showed no alteration in radiological density but re-ossifying bone in areas of re-vascularisation sometimes caused an absolute increase in radio-density. In an adjacent paper **Catto** studied late segmental collapse in 12 femoral heads and showed that it may not develop until $2^{1}/_{2}$ years after the fracture.

Epidemiology

Solomon L **Osteoporosis and fracture of the femoral neck in the South African Bantu** J Bone Joint Surg [Br] 1968;50-B:2–13

Gallagher JC, Melton LJ, Riggs BL, Bergstrathe E **The epidemiology of fractures of the proximal femur** Clin Orthop 1980;150:163–171

Boyce WJ, Vessey MP **Rising incidence of fracture of the proximal femur** Lancet 1985;I:150–151

Astrom J, Ahnqvist S, Beertema J, Jonsson B **Physical activity in women sustaining fracture of the neck of the femur** J Bone Joint Surg [Br] 1987; 69-B:381–383

Osteoporosis and Osteomalacia

Lane JM, Vigorita VJ **Current concepts review: osteoporosis** J Bone Joint Surg [Am] 1983;65-A:274–277

Wilton TJ, Hosking DJ, Pawley E, Stevens A, Harvey L **Osteomalacia and femoral neck fractures in the elderly** J Bone Joint Surg [Br] 1987;69-B: 388–390

Mortality

Jenson JS **Determining factors for the mortality following hip fractures** Injury 1984;15:411–414

Ions GK, Stevens J **Prediction of survival in patients with femoral neck fractures** J Bone Joint Surg [Br] 1987;69-B:384–387

The association of osteoporosis and fracture of the femoral neck has been deduced by epidemiological studies. **Solomon** showed that the fracture rate in the elderly Bantu is less than one-tenth of that in Western European population. **Gallagher** reported the incidence of fractures of the femoral neck over a 10-year period in the relatively small local population surrounding the Mayo Clinic. There was a doubling of fracture rate in each decade of life after the age of 50 in both men and women. It was estimated that by the age of 90, about one in three women and one in five men had suffered a fracture and this provided some idea of the enormous cost of this injury.

In the last decade, there has been a generalised increase in incidence of fracture of the proximal femur reported worldwide. **Boyce** compared the occurrence of this fracture in Oxford with that in a similar population 27 years previously. The incidence was found to have doubled in both sexes and the increase was apparent at all ages. **Astrom** submitted the hypothesis that physical inactivity during the fertile period of life in women increases the risk of sustaining a hip fracture later in life. He suggested that patients sustaining hip fractures between 60 and 70 years of age had been less active physically in their younger years than matched controls. A concise source of knowledge of the complex subject of osteoporosis is presented by **Lane**. The paper by **Wilton** has been included since he showed a 2% prevalence of osteomalacia in a series of over 1000 elderly patients with femoral neck fracture who were routinely screened by iliac crest biopsy. This suggested that osteomalacia is not a significant predisposing factor in the occurrence of this fracture.

Jenson studied 518 patients with hip fractures followed prospectively for three years. Life expectancy was found to be determined primarily by the patient's social dependence prior to fracture and secondarily, by the age of the patient.

There has been a renewed interest in what has been described as the biology of these fractures and this is reflected by **Ions** who performed a prospective study of factors which might help to predict mortality. The most important variable that had the greatest effect on the outcome was the mental ability of the patient as assessed by a score system. When the patients were demented and over the age of 85, the chances of survival was only 25%. This work questioned whether some patients are being over-treated.

Sub-capital Fractures

The Classics

Nicoll EA **Editorial: the unsolved fracture** J Bone Joint Surg [Br] 1963; 45-B:239–241

Garden RS **Malreduction and avascular necrosis in subcapital fractures of the femur** J Bone Joint Surg [Br] 1971;53-B:183–197

Barnes R, Brown JT, Garden RS, Nicoll EA **Subcapital fractures of the femur – a prospective review** J Bone Joint Surg [Br] 1976;58-B:2–24

The editorial written by **Nicoll** over 25 years ago provided a lucid and still pertinent summary of the debate in the management of this unsolved fracture. He presented a plea for the treatment of sub-capital fractures by selective conservatism rather than embarking on a policy of "wholesale decapitation". **Garden** described the accepted classification and the long-term results in a consecutive series of 322 healed sub-capital fractures. He emphasised the importance of a good reduction. The MRC trial by **Barnes** on the long-term investigation of 1503 sub-capital fractures is a classical study. Union occurred in almost all Garden Stage I and Stage II fractures treated by reduction and internal fixation but in only 67% of Stage III and Stage IV fractures. The age and physical state of the patient, the accuracy of reduction and the security of fixation had the greatest influence on non-union. The Smith-Peterson nail was found to be the least effective form of fixation in displaced fractures.

Treatment

Bentley GS **Impacted fractures of the neck of the femur** J Bone Joint Surg [Br] 1968;50-B:551–561

Sikorski JM, Barrington R **Internal fixation versus hemiarthroplasty for the displaced subcapital fracture of the femur – a prospective randomised study** J Bone Joint Surg [Br] 1981;63-B:357–361

Hunter GA **Should we abandon primary prosthetic replacement for fresh displaced fractures of the neck of the femur?** Clin Orthop 1980;152:158–161

Gingras MB, Clarke J, Evarts CM **Prosthetic replacement in femoral neck fractures** Clin Orthop 1980;152:147–157

Franklin A, Gallannaugh SC **The bi-articular hip prosthesis for fractures of the femoral neck – a preliminary report** Injury 1983;15:159–162

Stromqvist B **Hip fracture in rheumatoid arthritis** Acta Orthop Scand 1984;55:624–628

Avascular Necrosis

Stromqvist B **Femoral head vitality after intracapsular hip fracture** Acta Orthop Scand [Suppl] 1983;200:1–71

Linde F, Andersen E, Hvass I, Madsen F, Pallesen R **Avascular femoral head necrosis following fracture fixation** Injury 1986;17:159–163

Baksi DP **Treatment of post-traumatic avascular necrosis of the femoral head by multiple drilling and muscle-pedicle bone grafting: preliminary report** J Bone Joint Surg [Br] 1983;65-B:268–273

Bentley described the results of 70 patients who had had treatment for impacted fractures over a period of 12 years. 96% who were treated by primary internal fixation had good results.

Three papers have been included (**Sikorski, Hunter** and **Gingras**) which put forward with clear arguments the debate as to whether these fractures should be treated by internal fixation or by primary prosthetic replacement and, if the latter, by which approach? The authors gain the considerable impression that this is now still a matter of personal preference for the surgeon concerned. If prosthetic replacement is preferred, the paper of **Gingras** considered the benefits of the cemented prosthesis over the uncemented type.

Improved methods of internal fixation are now available compared with those used in Garden's classical work. All authors stress the necessity for an accurate anatomical reduction. Recent papers have endeavoured to clarify the benefits of different methods of internal fixation. For this reason we have included **Linde**'s article which discussed the effects on the head of the femur of fixation with either a dynamic hip screw or three AO screws. Some surgeons are now advocating the use of primary total hip replacement and for this reason, although the report is a preliminary one, the paper by **Franklin** has been included. **Stromqvist** discussed the treatment of hip fractures in rheumatoid arthritis and concluded these are best treated by primary prosthetic replacement.

In an attempt to study the blood supply **Stromqvist** examined 490 cases by intra-vital tetracycline labelling and radionuclide imaging. He concluded that this form of scintimetry performed within two weeks from femoral neck fracture can predict the outcome of the healing course with an accuracy of 91%. A prospective randomised trial of 104 consecutive patients with displaced fractures of the femoral neck treated with either a sliding screw plate or four AO cancellous bone screws was performed by **Linde**. The aim was to study the influence of the fixation device on the vascularity of the femoral head. The two treatment groups were comparable. There were significantly more avascular femoral heads in the sliding screw plate group than in those with the four AO cancellous bone screws. The treatment of avascular necrosis after a fracture of the neck of the femur especially in a younger patient is a major problem. We have therefore included a recent contribution by **Baksi** on the treatment of this complication by a muscle pedicle bone graft.

Stress Fractures

Devas MB **Stress fractures of the femoral neck** J Bone Joint Surg [Br] 1965; 47-B:728–738

Kaltas D-S **Stress fractures of the femoral neck in young adults: a report of seven cases** J Bone Joint Surg [Br] 1981;63-B:33–37

Twenty-five patients with stress fractures of the femoral neck are described by **Devas** in one of his early papers in 1965. Distinction was made between compression and transverse fractures and it was emphasised that the transverse stress fracture may become displaced and therefore must be recognised. **Kaltas** has drawn attention to stress fractures of the femoral neck in seven young adults. They were all recruits undergoing military training.

Inter-Trochanteric Fractures

The Classic

Evans EM **The treatment of trochanteric fractures of the femur** J Bone Joint Surg [Br] 1949;31-B:190–203

Epidemiology and Biomechanics

Jenson JS **Trochanteric fractures: an epidemiological, clinical and biomechanical study** Acta Orthop Scand [Suppl] 1988;52:1–100

Complications

Laros GS, Moore JF **Complications of fixation in inter-trochanteric fractures** Clin Orthop 1974;101:110–119

Treatment

James ETR, Hunter GA **The treatment of inter-trochanteric fractures: a review article** Injury 1983;14:421–431

Heyse-Moore GH, MacEachern AG, Jameson-Evans DC **The treatment of inter-trochanteric fractures of the femur – a comparison of the Richards screw plate with the Jewett nail plate** J Bone Joint Surg [Br] 1983;65-B:262–267

Esser MP, Kassab JY, Jones DHA **Trochanteric fractures of the femur: a randomised prospective trial comparing the Jewett nail plate with the dynamic hip screw** J Bone Joint Surg [Br] 1986;68-B:557–560

Bannister GC, Gibson AGF **Jewett nail plate or AO dynamic hip screw for trochanteric fractures? A randomised prospective controlled trial** J Bone Joint Surg [Br] 1983;65-B:218

Hall G, Ainscow DAP **Comparison of nail plate fixation and Ender's nailing for inter-trochanteric fractures** J Bone Joint Surg [Br] 1981;63-B:24–28

In a classic article published 40 years ago, **Evans** divided inter-trochanteric fractures into two types, the stable (72%) and the unstable (28%). **Jenson** studied 234 patients with a detailed analysis of the epidemiology, mortality and merits of various types of treatment. Sliding screw plate fixation is stronger than the Jewett; it is suitable especially for the unstable fracture since it allows secondary impaction and avoids technical failures of fixation. Complications of fixation have been studied by **Laros** based on an analysis of 244 surgically treated fractures. Valgus reduction reduced the risk of complications whereas a varus reduction increased the risk. Medial displacement osteotomy did not reduce the incidence of complications of fixation.

James reviewed all types of treatment, including the use of medial displacement osteotomy, valgus osteotomy and various medullary devices; the complications and mortality were discussed. A marginal preference is expressed for the use of the dynamic hip screw in two recent papers by **Esser** and **Heyse-Moore**. Mortality and morbidity were similar in the various types of fixation employed but it was considered that failures of stabilisation were less, both clinically and radiographically, in the patients treated by the various forms of dynamic hip screw. **Bannister** stated that the dynamic hip screw was three times as effective in allowing controlled collapse of the fracture. **Hall** considered that the use of Enders nails gave superior results in the treatment of trochanteric fractures. However, this subject is controversial particularly as knee problems may follow this operation. The authors have gained the impression that perhaps this method of fixation is less popular now than 10 years ago.

Hip Fractures in Children

Ratliff AHC **Fractures of the neck of the femur in children**. In: Salvati EA, ed. The hip. Proceedings of 9th Open scientific meeting 1981 St. Louis: CV Mosby, 1981:188–218

Canale ST **Traumatic dislocations and fracture-dislocations of the hip in children**. In: Salvati EA, ed. The hip. Proceedings of 9th Open scientific meeting 1981 St. Louis: CV Mosby, 1981:219–245

Leung PC, Lam SF **Long-term follow-up of children with femoral neck fractures** J Bone Joint Surg [Br] 1986;68-B:537–540

Ratliff AHC **Traumatic separation of the upper femoral epiphysis in young children** J Bone Joint Surg [Br] 1968;50-B:757–770

Fractures in the region of the hip are very rare but may have serious consequences. **Ratliff** has provided an analysis of the natural history and treatment of fractures of the neck of the femur in children based on a study of 168 patients. Complications are common and the injury is usually due to major violence. **Canale** has reviewed 49 patients with dislocations and fracture-dislocations of the hip in children. **Leung** showed an 83% incidence of radiographic abnormality in patients who had sustained a fracture of the femoral neck in childhood and observed for a minimum of 13 years after injury. One-quarter of these patients had pain, a limp or leg shortening. The characteristics of traumatic displacement of the upper femoral epiphysis in young children have been described by **Ratliff** based on a study of 13 cases. Separation of the upper femoral epiphysis is a serious injury which is likely to lead to permanent deformity.

Fractures of the Shaft of the Femur

Conservative Treatment

Buxton RA **The use of Perkins' traction in the treatment of femoral shaft fractures** J Bone Joint Surg [Br] 1981;63-B:362–366

Cast Bracing

Thomas TL, Meggitt BF **A comparative study of methods for treating fractures of the distal half of the femur** J Bone Joint Surg [Br] 1981;63-B:3–6

Meggitt BF, Juett DA, Smith JD **Cast bracing for fractures of the femoral shaft: a biomechanical and clinical study** J Bone Joint Surg [Br] 1981;63-B:12–23

Roper BA **Editorial: functional bracing of femoral fractures** J Bone Joint Surg [Br] 1981;63-B:1–2

Hardy AE **The treatment of femoral fractures by cast brace application and early ambulation: a prospective review of 106 patients** J Bone Joint Surg [Am] 1983;65-A:56–65

The treatment of fractures of the femoral shaft by traction may delay union and produce stiffness of the knee. **Buxton** described the technique of the Perkins' method of treatment and suggested that this has several advantages over other forms of traction. **Thomas** compared the results of different methods of treatment of fractures of the distal half of the femur and concluded that the cast brace provides a reliable method of treatment combining the advantages of non-operative management with early mobilisation. The mechanics of load-bearing were discussed by **Meggitt**. He considered that a brace functioned mainly as an anti-buckling hinged tube. **Roper**, in an editorial concluded that the cast brace method provided an excellent alternative to prolonged traction and internal fixation. **Hardy** presented a different opinion as a result of a prospective review of 106 patients. Problems of mal-alignment and shortening were discussed. He considered that the results of this method of treatment for comminuted fractures were "acceptable".

Intramedullary Nailing

Kuntscher G **Intramedullary surgical technique and its place in orthopaedic surgery. My present concept** J Bone Joint Surg [Am] 1965;47-A:809–818

Winquist RA, Hansen ST, Clawson DK **Closed intramedullary nailing of femoral fractures: a report of 520 cases** J Bone Joint Surg [Am] 1984;66-A:529–539

Kempf I, Grosse A, Beck G **Closed locked intramedullary nailing: its application to comminuted fractures of the femur** J Bone Joint Surg [Am] 1985;67-A:709–720

Zickel RE **An intramedullary fixation device for the proximal part of the femur – nine years experience** J Bone Joint Surg [Am] 1976;58-A:866–872

Kuntscher described the use of intramedullary fixation and his outstanding contribution is summarised in a paper published in 1965. **Winquist**, in a classic article, summarised treatment by intramedullary nailing in a report of 520 cases. The union rate was 99%. The incidence of infection was 0.9%. The operative technique is described with modifications with experience. **Kempf** discussed the treatment of severely comminuted fractures by closed locking in 59 cases. The aim is to control rotation or telescoping of the fragments by either static or dynamic locking. Operative technique and difficulties are discussed. **Zickel** summarised experience in the management of 84 non-pathological fractures in the sub-trochanteric region of the femur. There are useful comments concerning complications and limitations. The technique permitted early mobilisation of patients and afforded a high rate of union.

External Fixation

Dabezies EJ, D'Ambrosia R, Shoji H, Norris R, Murphy G **Fractures of the femoral shaft treated by external fixation with the Wagner device** J Bone Joint Surg [Am] 1984;66-A:360–364

Dabezies discussed the treatment of difficult and often complex femoral shaft fractures and described union occurring in 19 out of 20 cases. Chronic osteomyelitis did not develop in any of the patients.

In Children

Burton VW, Fordyce AJW **Immobilisation of femoral shaft fractures in children aged 2–10 years** Injury 1973;4:47–53

Sugi M, Cole WG **Early plaster treatment for fractures of the femoral shaft in childhood** J Bone Joint Surg [Br] 1987;69-B:743–745

Ziv I, Rang M **Treatment of femoral fracture in the child with a head injury** J Bone Joint Surg [Br] 1983;65-B:276–278

Edvardsen P, Syversen SM **Overgrowth of the femur after fracture of the shaft in childhood** J Bone Joint Surg [Br] 1976;58-B:339–342

Rang M **The femoral shaft** In: Children's fractures. 2nd edn Philadelphia: JB Lippincott, 1974:264–277

Reynolds DA **Growth changes in fractured long bones: a study of 126 children** J Bone Joint Surg [Br] 1981;63-B:83–88

Burton described a study of a late review of 84 children and compared the results of those treated on a splint with those treated in a plaster spica. There was little difference in the final result. Remodelling was more complete in the coronal than in the sagittal plane. **Sugi** advocated the early application of a hip spica in the management of these fractures. The method of treatment was simple, effective and dramatically reduced the cost of care. The special problems of management of children with an associated head injury were discussed by **Ziv** and open reduction and internal fixation proved an attractive solution. **Edvardsen** reviewed 26 children for differences of limb length seven to 10 years after injury. Two-thirds of the patients had overgrowth of the femur of one centimetre or more and shortening was well compensated by accelerated growth. The chapter in **Rang**'s book is included since general problems of management were discussed as was the use of gallows traction. **Reynolds** studied correction of shortening with growth after fractures of the long bones in 126 children. Within three months of injury, the rate of growth was at its maximum and was 38% in excess of normal. The greatest rate of growth occurred after injuries which resulted in overlap of the fragments.

With Associated Injuries

Veith RG, Winquist RA, Hansen ST Jr **Ipsilateral fractures of the femur and tibia: A report of 57 consecutive cases** J Bone Joint Surg [Am] 1984; 66-A:991–1002

Fraser RD, Hunter GA, Waddell JB **Ipsilateral fracture of the femur and tibia** J Bone Joint Surg [Br] 1978;60-B:510–515

Helal B, Skevis X **Unrecognised dislocation of the hip in fractures of the femoral shaft** J Bone Joint Surg [Br] 1967;49-B:293–299

Swiontkowski MC, Hansen ST, Kellam J **Ipsilateral fractures of the femoral neck and shaft: a treatment protocol** J Bone Joint Surg [Am] 1984;66-A: 260–268

Veith reported experience on the management of 57 consecutive cases of fractures of the femur and tibia. The multiple problems presented by these major injuries are discussed. Despite the serious nature of the local and sometimes associated injuries, good functional results can be achieved particularly when it is possible to internally fix both fractures. The paper by **Fraser** on the same subject has been included since the many complications including delayed union and non-union are emphasised. A cautionary warning of the 30% incidence of osteomyelitis in patients treated by internal fixation of both fractures is noted. **Helal** reported 14 cases where a dislocation of the hip had been missed in association with a fracture of the femoral shaft. He stressed the importance of awareness of dislocation where the fracture of the femur was transverse and the upper fragment adducted. **Swiontkowski** has been included since the special problems of management of a fracture of the femur in association with a fracture of the femoral neck are discussed.

Complicating Total Hip Replacement

Barrington TW, Johansson JE, McBroom RJ **Fractures of the femur complicating total hip replacement** In: Ling RSM, ed. Complications of total hip replacement Edinburgh, etc: Churchill Livingstone, 1984:30–40

Cooke PH, Newman JH **Fractures of the femur in relation to cemented hip prostheses** J Bone Joint Surg [Br] 1988;70-B:386–389

There is now a growing awareness of the incidence of fractures complicating total hip replacement and these may occur both during operation and later. **Barrington** analysed 36 such fractures. They are conveniently classified into three types and predisposing causes and results of treatment discussed. Intra-operative fracture can usually be avoided by pre-operative assessment and care during surgery. A post-operative fracture of the shaft frequently needs radical and determined surgery. **Cooke** reviewed the results of 75 fractures of the proximal femoral shaft in the presence of a cemented femoral prosthesis. They are divided into four types. The controversy concerning management of these various types is debated.

Supracondylar Fractures of the Femur in the Adult

Neer CS, Grantham SA, Shelton ML **Supracondylar fractures of the adult femur: a study of 110 cases** J Bone Joint Surg [Am] 1967;49-A:591–613

Sarmiento A, Latta LL **Fractures of the femur.** In: Closed functional treatment of fractures Berlin, etc: Springer-Verlag, 1981:297–338

Schatzker J, Horn G, Waddell J **The Toronto experience with the supracondylar fracture of the femur: 1966 – 1972** Injury 1974;6:113–128

Schatzker J **Supracondylar fractures of the femur** In: Schatzker J, Tile M, ed. The rationale of operative fracture care Berlin, etc: Springer-Verlag, 1987: 255–273

A supracondylar fracture, often comminuted and sometimes involving the articular surface of the knee joint, may present formidable problems of management especially in the younger adult. The four papers selected reflect the recent considerable change in the approach to treatment. **Neer** described in 1967 the results which may be expected where conservative treatment is preferred and this may be indicated in the older patient with osteoporotic bone. Only 52% of patients obtained a result classified as satisfactory. Cast bracing described by **Sarmiento** allows earlier ambulation. Precise details of application are illustrated.

Schatzker in 1974 summed up the Toronto experience. Strict criteria were applied in the evaluation of results and the failures of both the surgically and conservatively treated groups analysed. Those treated with the AO method had 75% good or excellent results. It was, however, stressed that the operation has to be performed very carefully to obtain a good result with no problem of union, valgus or varus and reasonable movement. This theme is amplified in the recent publication in 1987. Absolute and relative indications for surgery are discussed and details of operative technique described. A classification is illustrated, type C being comminuted and involving the articular surface. In any supracondylar segment with bone loss or severe comminution, bone grafting is recommended. Methylmethacrylate may be useful in patients with osteoporosis. **Schatzker** concluded "the only patients in whom a poor result can be accepted are those with C3 fractures in which the articular portion of the fracture is irreconstructible".

Supracondylar Fractures of the Femur in the Child

Rang M **Supracondylar fractures in children** In: Children's fractures. 2nd edn Philadelphia: JB Lippincott, 1983;277–280

Lombardo SJ, Harvey JP **Fractures of the distal femoral epiphyses. Factors influencing prognosis. A review of 34 cases** J Bone Joint Surg [Am] 1977; 59-A:742–751

Riseborough EJ, Barrett IR, Shapiro F **Growth disturbances following distal femoral physeal fracture-separations** J Bone Joint Surg [Am] 1983;65-A: 885–893

Rang has provided a short review of this subject dividing injuries where there is separation of the distal femoral epiphysis into the extension and valgus types. It is now appreciated that not all epiphyseal separations continue to grow normally. **Lombardo** studied 34 fractures through this distal epiphyseal plate followed for an average of four years and found limb length discrepancy of two centimetres or more in 36%, and that approximately the same number developed either a valgus or varus deformity. In a collected series of 66 distal femoral physeal fracture-separations, **Riseborough** has drawn attention to the considerable problems of abnormal growth that may occur. The complications listed are not necessarily a true reflection of the frequency following such fractures but growth problems correlated well with the severity of trauma and were seen in each of the Salter–Harris types. The paper is a useful reminder of the importance of these complications.

Soft Tissue Injuries of the Knee

Anatomy and Biomechanics

Jackson JP **Surgical anatomy** In: Jackson JP, Waugh W, ed. Surgery of the knee London: Chapman and Hall, 1984:3–32

Burstein AH **Biomechanics of the knee** In: Insall JN, ed. Surgery of the knee Edinburgh, etc: Churchill Livingstone, 1984:21–39

Butler DL, Noyes FR, Grood ES **Ligamentous restraints to anterior-posterior draw in the human knee. A biomechanical study** J Bone Joint Surg [Am] 1980;62-A:259–270

Grood ES, Noyes FR, Butler DL, Suntay WJ **Ligamentous and capsular restraints preventing straight medial and lateral laxity in intact human cadaver knees** J Bone Joint Surg [Am] 1981;63-A:1257–1269

Assessment

Simonsen O, Jenson J, Mouritsen P, Lauritzen J **The accuracy of clinical examination of injury of the knee joint** Injury 1984;16:96–101

Jackson RW, Abe I **The role of arthroscopy in the management of disorders of the knee: an analysis of 200 consecutive examinations** J Bone Joint Surg [Br] 1972;54-B:310–322

Ireland J, Trickey EL, Stoker DJ **Arthroscopy and arthrography of the knee: a critical review** J Bone Joint Surg [Br] 1980;62-B:3–6

Casteleyn PP, Handelberg F, Opdecam P **Traumatic haemarthrosis of the knee** J Bone Joint Surg [Br] 1988;70-B:404–406

Dandy DJ **Arthroscopy of the knee. A diagnostic colour atlas** London, etc: Butterworth, 1984

Jackson provided a clear review of the anatomy and although **Burstein**'s work is primarily directed towards total knee replacement, it summarised the biomechanics of the knee. The papers by **Butler** and **Grood** demonstrated in cadaveric knee experiments the primary and secondary ligamentous restraints to antero-posterior, medial and lateral movement. Their work explained how isolated ligamentous injuries may be masked in clinical examination, at least in the early stages and that for significant disruption of the knee, there is often a combination of injuries.

Simonsen's paper emphasised that the acutely injured knee is difficult to assess by simple clinical examination. The use of the arthroscope is now accepted. **Jackson** in 1979 described his first five years' experience and found it had been of benefit in 75%

of patients. **Ireland** emphasised the complementary role of arthrography and stated that by using both investigations the correct diagnosis could be achieved in 98% of patients. **Casteleyn** assessed patients presenting with traumatic haemarthrosis and found that 99 out of 100 patients had significant pathology. The study confirmed the importance of an acute traumatic haemarthrosis even in patients who were not athletes. There is a considerable literature on arthroscopic techniques and **Dandy** has provided an extremely well illustrated review of the subject.

Injuries of the Meniscus

Allen PR, Denham RA, Swan AV **Late degenerative changes after menisectomy. Factors affecting the knee after operation** J Bone Joint Surg [Br] 1984;66-B:666–671

Northmore-Ball MD, Dandy DJ, Jackson RW **Arthroscopic, open partial, and total menisectomy: a comparative study** J Bone Joint Surg [Br] 1983; 65-B:400–404

Scott GA, Jolly BL, Henning CE **Combined posterior incision and arthroscopic intra-articular repair of the meniscus** J Bone Joint Surg [Am] 1986;68-A:847–861

A more cautious approach to menisectomy should now be adopted following **Allen**'s paper reviewing its late effects in 210 patients with follow-up of between 10 and 22 years; he found 7% with significant symptoms and signs of joint degeneration and there were radiological changes in a further 11%. With a shorter follow-up, **Northmore-Ball** demonstrated the advantages of arthroscopic partial menisectomy over an open procedure. The alternative of preservation of the meniscus has been described by **Scott**. He reviewed the results of surgical repair of 178 menisci and found 61% had healed completely and in 92% of cases, the meniscus was stable.

Acute Ligament Injuries

Hughston JC, Andrews JR, Cross MJ, Moschi A **Classification of the knee ligament instabilities. Part I. The medial compartment and cruciate ligaments** J Bone Joint Surg [Am] 1976;58-A:159–172

Hughston JC, Andrews JR, Cross MJ, Moschi A **Classification of the knee ligament instabilities. Part II. The lateral compartment** J Bone Joint Surg [Am] 1976;58-A:173–179

McDaniel WJ, Dameron TB **Untreated ruptures of the anterior cruciate ligament: a follow-up study** J Bone Joint Surg [Am] 1980;62-A:696–705

Kannus P, Jarvinen M **Conservatively treated tears of the anterior cruciate ligament: long-term results** J Bone Joint Surg [Am] 1987;69-A:1007–1012

Sandberg R, Balkfors B, Nilsson B, Westlin N **Operative versus non-operative treatment of recent injuries to the ligaments of the knee. A prospective randomised study** J Bone Joint Surg [Am] 1987;69-A:1120–1126

Noyes FR, McGinniss GH **Controversy about the treatment of the knee with anterior cruciate laxity** Clin Orthop 1985;198:61–76

Trickey EL **Rupture of the posterior cruciate ligament of the knee** J Bone Joint Surg [Br] 1968;50-B:334–341

Dandy DJ, Pussey RJ **The long-term results of unrepaired tears of the posterior cruciate ligament** J Bone Joint Surg [Br] 1982;64-B:92–94

A summary of the diagnosis and treatment of ligamentous injuries of the knee is difficult. **Hughston** classified these injuries in two large papers in 1976. However, controversy still exists concerning the contribution made by different structures in maintaining stability of the knee and also the value of conservative or surgical treatment.

Many articles have been written concerning the anterior cruciate deficient knee. **McDaniel** originally outlined the problems and, since, several authors have described the increase in degenerative changes that occur with advancing years. **Kannus** has highlighted the difference in outcome between the partially and completely ruptured anterior cruciate ligament treated conservatively. In those patients with a completely ruptured ligaments, there was instability and early degenerative osteoarthritis. Later reconstruction was frequently necessary. This was in contrast to those with a partially ruptured ligament. In a prospective randomised trial of 200 patients, **Sandberg** presented the results of ligament injuries treated conservatively or surgically. Injuries to the medial ligaments did not benefit from surgery. The results of ruptured medial ligament were not significantly different whether treated conservatively or operatively. Similarly, for anterior cruciate ligament tears, there was no significant difference in those treated by the two methods.

We have not attempted to include the many different types of repair or reconstruction that have been advocated in the treatment of patients with deficiency of the anterior cruciate. **Noyes** summarised the controversy and this paper provides a current review of the subject.

Seventeen cases of knee injury are described by **Trickey** in which the predominant lesion was rupture of the posterior cruciate ligament. Seven were treated conservatively and ten by surgical repair. Early surgical repair is recommended for complete rupture and a precise technique described.

Based on a study of a group of 20 patients with ruptures of the posterior cruciate ligament, **Dandy** suggested that many patients with this insufficiency have a good functional result and that the place of routine repair of such injuries should be questioned.

Chronic Instability

Insall JN **Chronic instability of the knee** In: Surgery of the knee Edinburgh, etc: Churchill Livingstone, 1984:295–352

The well illustrated chapter by **Insall** on chronic instability discussed the diagnosis of this condition and the methods of testing for different types of instability. The types of operation that have been recommended for this problem are fully described. The subject is complex and the authors have preferred this chapter to a number of separate articles. Long-term results are still necessary to compare the value of each technique.

Dislocations of the Knee

Conservative Treatment

Taylor AR, Arden GP, Rainey HA **Traumatic dislocation of the knee. A report of 43 cases with special reference to conservative treatment** J Bone Joint Surg [Br] 1972;54-B:96–102

Operative Treatment

Meyers MH, Harvey JP **Traumatic dislocation of the knee joint. A study of 18 cases** J Bone Joint Surg [Am] 1971;53-A:16–29

These injuries are rare and individual experience small. **Taylor** discussed the results of management of 42 cases largely treated by conservative methods. Conservative treatment of 26 dislocations yielded surprisingly good results with regard to stability, absence of pain and range of flexion. The paper by **Meyers** advocated early repair of all capsular tears and interrupted ligaments including the posterior cruciate ligament. The results in 18 patients were discussed. The authors suggest the reader should be aware of the relatively small knowledge available and decide which philosophy he will adopt. Complications are discussed. Major vascular damage is the most serious and it is of some interest that in the combined series there were eight cases out of a total of 60.

Fractures of the Patella

Excision

Scott JC **Fractures of the patella** J Bone Joint Surg [Br] 1949;31-B:76–81

Wilkinson J **Fractures of the patella treated by total excision: a long-term follow-up** J Bone Joint Surg [Br] 1977;59-B:352–354

Treatment of Comminuted Fracture

Bostman O, Kiviluoto O, Nirhamo J **Comminuted displaced fractures of the patella** Injury 1982;13:196–202

Technique of Fixation

Muller ME, Allgower M, Schneider R, Willenegger H **Manual of internal fixation**. 2nd edn Berlin, etc: Springer-Verlag, 1979:248–253

The management of fractures of the patella is perhaps more debatable than sometimes appreciated in the standard textbooks. **Wilkinson** discussed a long follow-up of patients who had total excision and stated that 40% had poor results. He referred to an article by **Scott** in 1949 where many patients had a significant disability and only 5% reported a normal knee. The AO Manual (**Muller**) describes the technique for stable fixation of fractures of this bone, including those which are comminuted. **Bostman**'s paper has been included as reflecting a trend towards retention of the patella wherever possible and emphasising the difficulty of making a choice between excision and internal fixation.

Dislocations of the Patella

Acute

Cofield RH, Bryan RS **Acute dislocation of the patella. Results of conservative treatment** J Trauma 1977;17:526–531

Recurrent

Heywood AWB **Recurrent dislocation of the patella. A study of its pathology and treatment in 106 knees** J Bone Joint Surg [Br] 1961;43-B:508–517

Insall J, Goldberg V, Salvati E **Recurrent dislocation and the high-riding patella** Clin Orthop 1972;88:67–69

Hampson WGJ, Hill P **Late results of transfer of the tibial tubercle for recurrent dislocation of the patella** J Bone Joint Surg [Br] 1975;57-B:209–213

Hughston JC, Walsh WM **Proximal and distal reconstruction of the extensor mechanism for patella subluxation** Clin Orthop 1979;144:36–42

Habitual

Bergman NR, Williams PF **Habitual dislocations of the patella in flexion** J Bone Joint Surg [Br] 1988;70-B:415–419

The article by **Cofield** presented a series of 50 cases of acute dislocation of the patella followed for a minimum of five years. In nearly half (44%) at least one further dislocation occurred and in one-quarter sufficient symptoms developed to warrant later reconstructive surgery after the first episode.

The literature on recurrent subluxation and dislocation concentrates on methods of surgical treatment. **Heywood** described the pathological changes in the patella and considered that for young adults, where degenerative changes were not severe, transplant of the tibial tubercle gave the best results. This operation is contra-indicated in children because it may result in a recurvatum deformity. Based on an analysis of 77 patients, **Insall** showed that a high-riding patella is usually found in recurrent dislocation. A study of the position of the patella may provide a guide as to whether distal advancement of the tibial tubercle is necessary. **Hampson** studied the late results of the Hauser operation with special reference to the development of osteoarthritis. Forty-four surgically treated knees were examined to an average of 16 years after operation. There was a high incidence of osteoarthritis (70%). Whilst the Hauser operation prevented further dislocation, it did not prevent the development of osteoarthritis. The study by **Hughston** is important as it recorded 700 cases of disabling patella subluxation of which more than 50% recovered well by conservative means. He described combined proximal and distal reconstruction in a large series of patients with good and excellent results in 70%. This operation was advised and detailed technique described.

Bergman reviewed 35 patients with habitual dislocation of the patella in flexion. Quadriceps lengthening is considered an essential part of treatment and must be performed proximally. The vastus medialis however is rarely affected.

Dislocation of the Proximal Tibiofibular Joint

Ogden JA **Subluxation and dislocation of the proximal tibiofibular joint** J Bone Joint Surg [Am] 1974;56-A:145–154

Ogden found four types of instability or disruption of the proximal tibiofibular joint in a series of 43 cases. Early diagnosis was missed in about one-third. Most responded satisfactorily to closed reduction. This paper provides a useful reference to a rare injury.

Fractures of the Tibial Plateau

Conservative Treatment

Apley AG **Fractures of the lateral tibial condyle treated by skeletal traction and early mobilisation: a review of 60 cases with special reference to the long-term results** J Bone Joint Surg [Br] 1956;38-B:699–708

Lansinger O, Bergman B, Korner L, Andersson GBJ **Tibial condylar fractures: a 20 year follow-up** J Bone Joint Surg [Am] 1986;68-A:13–19

Sarmiento A, Kinman PB, Latta LL **Fractures of the proximal tibia and tibial condyles: a clinical and laboratory comparative study** Clin Orthop 1979;145:136–145

Operative Treatment

Schatzker J, McBroom R, Bruce D **The tibial plateau fracture: the Toronto experience 1968–1975** Clin Orthop 1979;138:94–104

Review Article

Schatzker J **Fractures of the tibial plateau** In: Schatzker J, Tile M, ed. The rationale of operative fracture care Berlin, etc: Springer-Verlag, 1987:279–295

Apley described a method of skeletal traction with early mobilisation for these injuries. The results were described as satisfactory and there was no evidence of late deterioration of the joint. A 20-year follow-up of 204 patients is described by **Lansinger**. Ninety per cent of the patients achieved an excellent or good result. It was recommended that depressed fractures with an unstable knee should be treated surgically.

    Sarmiento discussed the management of 106 fractures in a specialised clinic. It was concluded that selected condylar and proximal tibial shaft fractures could be success-fully treated by non surgical means but where incongruity of the articular surface has to be accepted, restoration of motion is essential. Where it is intact, the mechanical role of the fibula is emphasised.

The Toronto experience over a number of years is outlined by **Schatzker** and, despite the severity of the injury, 80% of those patients who came to surgery, obtained a satisfactory result.

Schatzker has recently classified these injuries into six different types and dis-cussed in detail the operative technique. He considered that the result of a failed open reduction and internal fixation is always worse than the result of failed closed treatment. A detailed algorithm is suggested for the management of different types of case and at different ages. There is a current trend towards internal fixation of these fractures particularly where there is instability.

Fractures of the Tibia

The Classics

Ellis H **The speed of healing after fracture of the tibial shaft** J Bone Joint Surg [Br] 1958;40-B:42–46

Nicoll EA **Fractures of the tibial shaft: a survey of 705 cases** J Bone Joint Surg [Br] 1964;46-B:373–387

In 1958 **Ellis** reported the results of a study of 343 tibial shaft fractures in adults which were proceeding to union. Where the severity of injury (as assessed by the degree of displacement, of comminution and compound wounding) was classified as major, delayed union occurred in 60%.

Nicoll described the results that can be expected from conservative immobilisation in a long leg plaster cast. He coined the term "personality of the fracture" and concluded that no case has yet been made for internal fixation as the method of choice in the treatment of this fracture.

Cast Bracing

Sarmiento A **A functional below-the-knee brace for tibial fractures: a report on its use in 135 cases** J Bone Joint Surg [Am] 1970;52-A:295–311

Internal Fixation: Plating

Ruedi T, Webb JK, Allgower M **Experience with the dynamic compression plate (DCP) in 418 recent fractures of the tibial shaft** Injury 1976;7:252–257

Christensen J, Jorgen G, Rosendahl S **Fractures of the shaft of the tibia treated with AO compression osteo-synthesis** Injury 1982;13:307–314

Internal Fixation: Intramedullary Nailing

Bone LB, Johnson KD **Treatment of tibial fractures by reaming and intramedullary nailing** J Bone Joint Surg [Am] 1986;68-A:877–887

Sarmiento has described how bracing can allow early mobilisation of joints. His biomechanical and clinical studies indicated few complications with early weight bearing. The vast majority of tibial fractures will heal with non-operative treatment.

The AO group have stressed the poor functional results that may be obtained by non-operative treatment and they have placed open reduction and rigid internal fixation on a firm scientific basis. They believe that failure of surgical treatment is mainly the result of poor technique. With stable internal fixation, plaster disease is eliminated.

In 1976 the results of a consecutive series of 435 fresh fractures of the tibial shaft internally fixed by a dynamic compression plate were described by **Ruedi**. Later, **Christensen** discussed experience with the treatment of 96 displaced fractures of the tibia by AO internal fixation. Of these, 40% were open fractures. It was considered that rigid internal fixation should be the method of treatment for all displaced fractures of the shaft of the tibia and it was advocated as an urgent procedure especially in open fractures.

Intramedullary nailing has been advocated by some surgeons as it avoids exposure of the fracture and allows early weight bearing. **Bone** described the newer locking techniques, thus allowing use in comminuted and more proximally or distally displaced fractures. The treatment of non-union is also illustrated by this technique.

External Fixation and Open Fractures

Velazco A, Fleming LL **Open fractures of the tibia treated by the Hoffman external fixator** Clin Orthop 1983;180:125–132

Behrens F, Searls K **External fixation of the tibia – basic concepts and prospective evaluation** J Bone Joint Surg [Br] 1986;68-B:246–254

Velazco A, Whitesides TE, Fleming LL **Open fractures of the tibia treated with the Lottes nail** J Bone Joint Surg [Am] 1983;65-A:879–885

James ETR, Gruss JS **Closure of osteomyelitic and traumatic defects of the leg by muscle and musculocutaneous flaps** J Trauma 1983;23:411–419

Lange RH, Bach AW, Hansen ST, Johansen KH **Open tibial fractures with associated vascular injuries: prognosis for limb salvage** J Trauma 1985;25:203–208

Two papers have been included on the use of external fixation in the treatment of open fractures. **Velazco** described the results of treatment of a prospective study of 40 patients. The wounds were all left open and classified as Gustilo types II and III. **Behrens** noted the high rate of complications with external fixation. He stressed basic principles that govern the optimal use of these devices and that by following them, the majority of complications can be eliminated. **Velazco** discussed the treatment of fifty consecutive open fractures with immediate intramedullary Lottes nail fixation and debridement and irrigation of the wound. The rate of infection was 6%. **James** discussed the recent advances and methods of treatment of skin loss by appropriate muscle and musculocutaneous flaps based on an experience of 17 difficult cases. It was concluded that these methods offer a safe and reliable technique for cover of defects of the leg from both trauma and chronic osteomyelitis. The management of open tibial fractures with associated vascular injuries was described by **Lange**. Crush injuries, segmental tibial fractures and re-vascularisation delays of greater than six hours were associated with a bad outcome. There was an amputation rate of 60% in 23 severe injuries.

Non-Union

Reckling FW, Waters CH **Treatment of non-unions of fractures of the tibial diaphysis by postero-lateral cortical cancellous bone grafting** J Bone Joint Surg [Am] 1980;62-A:936–941

Bassett CAL, Mitchell SN, Gaston SR **Treatment of un-united tibial diaphyseal fractures with pulsing electromagnetic fields** J Bone Joint Surg [Am] 1981; 63-A:511–523

Chacha PB, Ahmed M, Daruwalla JS **Vascular pedicle graft of the ipsilateral fibula for non-union of the tibia with a large defect – an experimental and clinical study** J Bone Joint Surg [Br] 1981;63-B:244–253

Reckling outlined the results of bone grafting in the treatment of 44 consecutive tibial diaphyseal fractures with non-union. A postero-lateral approach is advocated to avoid wound problems with the anterior approach. **Bassett** stated that the overall success rate in the treatment of 177 un-united tibial fractures with pulsating electromagnetic fields was 87%. **Chacha** provided a full description of the operative technique and complications when using a vascularised fibula graft in 11 patients with large tibial defects. It will be recalled that both Muller and Rosen have discussed the treatment of delayed and non-union and references to their papers are included in the general section on this subject.

Ipsi-lateral Fractures of the Tibia and Femur

Veith RG, Winquist RA, Hansen TR Jr **Ipsi-lateral fractures of the femur and tibia: a report of 57 consecutive cases** J Bone Joint Surg [Am] 1984; 66-A:991–1002

Fraser RD, Hunter GA, Waddell JB **Ipsi-lateral fracture of the femur and tibia** J Bone Joint Surg [Br] 1978;60-B:510–515

Veith reported experience on the management of 57 consecutive cases of fractures of the femur and tibia. The multiple problems presented by these major injuries are discussed. Despite the serious nature of the local and sometimes associated injuries, good functional results can be achieved particularly when it is possible to internally fix both fractures. The paper by **Fraser** on the same subject has been included since the many complications including delayed union and non-union are stressed. A cautionary warning of the 30% incidence of osteomyelitis in patients treated by internal fixation of both fractures is noted.

Review Article

Tile M **Fractures of the tibia** In: Schatzker J, Tile M, ed. The rationale of operative fracture care Berlin, etc: Springer-Verlag, 1987:297–340

There are many aspects of the management of fractures of the tibia which continue to be subjects of considerable debate and controversy. **Tile** has recently produced a comprehensive chapter on this subject which presents a thoughtful review of these controversies.

Ankle Fractures

Classification

Heim U, Pfeiffer KM **Malleolar fractures** In: Internal fixation of small fractures. Technique recommended by the AO-ASIF Group. 3rd edn. Berlin, etc: Springer-Verlag, 1988:286–297

Surgical Treatment

Yablon IG, Heller FG, Shouse L **The key role of the lateral malleolus in displaced fractures of the ankle** J Bone Joint Surg [Am] 1977;59-A:169–173

Pankovich AM **Fractures of the fibula proximal to the distal tibiofibular syndesmosis** J Bone Joint Surg [Am] 1978;60-A:221–229

De Souza LJ, Gustilo RB, Meyer TJ **Results of operative treatment of displaced external rotation – abduction fractures of the ankle** J Bone Joint Surg [Am] 1985;67-A:1066–1074

Ruedi TP, Allgower M **The operative treatment of intra-articular fractures of the lower end of the tibia** Clin Orthop 1979;138:105–110

Fractures in the Elderly

Beauchamp CG, Clay NR, Thexton PW **Displaced ankle fractures in patients over 50 years of age** J Bone Joint Surg [Br] 1983;65-B:329–332

Ali MS, McLaren CAN, Rouholamin E, O'Connor BT **Ankle fractures in the elderly. Non-operative or operative treatment** J Orthop Trauma 1988;1:275–280

Comparison of Operative and Conservative Treatment

Hughes JL, Weber H, Willenegger H, Kuner EH **Evaluation of ankle fractures: non-operative and operative treatment** Clin Orthop 1979;138:111–119

Rowley DI, Norris SH, Duckworth T **A prospective trial comparing operative and manipulative treatment of ankle fractures** J Bone Joint Surg [Br] 1986;68-B:610–613

Long-Term Follow-Up

Bauer M, Jonsson K, Nilsson B **Thirty-year follow-up of ankle fractures** Acta Orthop Scand 1985;56:103–106

Tri-plane Fractures

Spiegel PG, Mast JW, Cooperman DR, Laros GS **Tri-plane fractures of the distal tibial epiphysis** Clin Orthop 1984;188:74–89

Review Article

Tile M **Fractures of the ankle** In: Schatzker J, Tile M, ed. The rationale of operative fracture care Berlin, etc: Springer-Verlag, 1987: 371–405

The Danis–Weber classification is clearly outlined in the AO manual (**Heim**) and is now the accepted method of classification of ankle fractures. The more complex Lauge–Hansen classification relates to the mechanism of injury and its understanding facilitates closed reduction. The former classification is more orientated towards open reduction and internal fixation.

Yablon emphasised that the relationship of the talus to the lateral malleolus is crucial. Anatomical reduction of the fibula is essential for satisfactory results and prevention of late degenerative arthritis. **Pankovich** described all three different types of fracture of the fibula above the level of the inferior tibiofibular syndesmosis and considered that these different types demonstrated the likely mechanisms of injury. **De Souza** described a follow-up of 150 displaced ankle fractures which had been openly reduced and internally fixed. These papers stressed the importance of restoring fibula length and suggested that up to 2mm of displacement of the fibula may be accepted. It was not necessary to fix a fracture of the posterior malleolus providing less than 25% of the articular surface is involved. The operative treatment of difficult intra-articular distal tibial fractures is discussed by **Ruedi**. Good results (70%) can be achieved in expert hands.

Beauchamp considered the controversial problem of operating on older patients and advocated conservative management. **Ali** disagreed with this opinion; a high proportion of poor results in a conservatively treated group correlated well with mal-union and non-union.

During the last decade there has been a marked trend towards internal fixation of the unstable ankle fractures and this is exemplified by the paper by **Hughes** from the AO school, discussing results of treatment. In contrast, the authors have recently been stimulated by the article by **Rowley** which suggested that the immediate outcome between two similar groups of patients treated by the AO technique and by conservative treatment is not different, at least in the early recovery period. This article is inserted to highlight a possible controversy.

The paper by **Bauer** is included since it is one of the few long-term follow-up studies of injuries of the ankle. A reference has been included to tri-plane fractures by **Spiegel** since it is thought that readers should be aware of interest in this complicated injury in the lower tibial epiphysis in growing children. The natural history, classification, assessment of stability and management of ankle fractures has recently been reviewed in a separate chapter by **Tile**. Special problems, such as open ankle fractures, injuries in the elderly and fibular lengthening for mal-union are also discussed.

Injuries of the Lateral Ligament of the Ankle

Evans GA, Frenyo SD **The stress-tenogram in the diagnosis of ruptures of the lateral ligament of the ankle** J Bone Joint Surg [Br] 1979;61-B:347–351

Evans GA, Hardcastle P, Frenyo SD **Acute rupture of the lateral ligament of the ankle: to suture or not to suture?** J Bone Joint Surg [Br] 1984;66-B:209–212

Sefton GK, George J, Fitton JM, McMullen H **Reconstruction of the anterior talofibular ligament for the treatment of the unstable ankle** J Bone Joint Surg [Br] 1979;61-B:352–354

Three references illustrate debate on the diagnosis and management of ruptures of the lateral ligament of the ankle. It is not easy to differentiate between those ankles classified as stable and unstable and **Evans** described a radiological technique for the investigation of injuries to the lateral ligament of the ankle by stress tenograms. He combined the information previously provided by stress radiographs and the peroneal tenogram and considered that a high degree of diagnostic accuracy had been confirmed at operative repair in a group of 32 patients. In a later paper, **Evans** described the results of a prospective study to assess the value of operative repair of acute rupture of the lateral ligament of the ankle. He concluded there was no evidence that operative repair offered significant benefit. An operative technique with results is described by **Sefton** for the use of a free tendon graft to reconstruct the anterior talo-fibular ligament in patients with chronic instability of the ankle after injury. The operation would appear to be more simple than previously described methods and has the advantage of not restricting movement at the sub-talar level.

Rupture of the Achilles Tendon

Nistor L **Surgical and non-surgical treatment of Achilles tendon rupture: a prospective randomised study** J Bone Joint Surg [Am] 1981;63-A;394–399

Carden DG, Noble J, Chalmers J, Lunn P, Ellis J **Rupture of the calcaneal tendon. The early and late management** J Bone Joint Surg [Br] 1987;69-B: 416–420

Barnes MJ, Hardy AE **Delayed reconstruction of the calcaneal tendon** J Bone Joint Surg [Br] 1986;68-B:121–124

Controversy exists as to whether in the acute stage ruptures of the Achilles tendon should be repaired. **Nistor** presented a prospective randomised study comparing the value of operative and conservative treatment. Only minor differences were noted between the final results of the two groups and it was concluded that non-surgical treatment offers advantages over surgical treatment. **Carden** reviewed the results of treatment of 106 patients. The incidence of major complications was higher after operation than in those treated conservatively but patients who were treated more than one week after injury had an inferior result when treated conservatively. It was therefore recommended that calcaneal tendon rupture be treated conservatively when diagnosed within 48 hours of injury but by operation when diagnosis has been delayed for more than one week. **Barnes** studied the results of surgical treatment of 13 patients where the tendon rupture was diagnosed more than four weeks after injury. The results suggested that late reconstruction of a ruptured calcaneal tendon is a worthwhile procedure.

Fractures of the Talus

The Classic

Coltart WD "Aviators astragalus" J Bone Joint Surg [Br] 1952;34-B:545–566

Biomechanics

Peterson L, Romanis B, Dahlberg E **Fracture of the collum talus: an experimental study** J Biomech 1976;9:277–279

Blood Supply

Mulfinger GL, Trueta J **The blood supply of the talus** J Bone Joint Surg [Br] 1970;52-B:160–167

Classification and Operative Treatment

Grob D, Simpson LA, Weber BG, Bray T **Operative treatment of displaced talus fractures** Clin Orthop 1985;199:88–96

Tile M **Fractures of the talus** In: Schatzker J, Tile M, ed. The rationale of operative fracture care Berlin, etc: Springer-Verlag, 1987:407–432

Long-Term Results

Canale ST, Kelly FB **Fractures of the neck of the talus. Long-term evaluation of 71 cases** J Bone Joint Surg [Am] 1978;60-A:143–156

Fractures of the talus have been associated with aviator injuries and **Coltart** studied those that occurred during World War II in the Royal Air Force. He classified 228 fractures, discussed the possible mechanisms of injury and also the complications including infection, avascular necrosis and arthritis of adjacent joints.

More recently the possible mechanism of injury has been investigated by **Peterson** on cadaveric specimens. He found that a fracture of the talus could be experimentally produced when a foot was struck from below and braced both in front and behind the ankle joint. It could not be produced when the same force was used and the flaccid forefoot was dorsiflexed.

Mulfinger has described in detail the blood supply and discussed clinical applications. Most fractures of the neck of the talus do not cause avascular necrosis of the body. Avascular necrosis after simple fractures of the neck must imply unrecognised serious soft tissue damage. Triple arthrodesis also interferes with the blood supply to this bone.

Grob used the classification of Marti and Weber and reviewed 41 cases. He described the operative method of reduction and fixation of the fracture with a single screw. **Tile** has recently updated knowledge on this subject and particularly discussed surgical technique, skin incisions and methods of internal fixation.

Canale reviewed 71 cases and stressed that avascular necrosis, although increasing in frequency with the greater severity of the fracture, did not necessarily lead to a poor clinical result. This complication occurred in 52%. He also reported that even if the result of primary treatment was poor, secondary salvage operations were usually successful.

Sub-Talar Dislocation of the Foot

DeLee JC, Curtis R **Sub-talar dislocation of the foot** J Bone Joint Surg [Am] 1982;64-A:433–437

Seventeen cases of this rare injury were presented. The treatment programmes and results were outlined and the factors associated with a poor result discussed. Lateral dislocations were prone to poor results due to the frequency of open injuries and associated fractures.

Fractures of the Calcaneum

The Classic

Essex-Lopresti P **The mechanism, reduction technique and results in fractures of the os calcis** Br J Surg 1951;39:395–419

An Atlas

Warrick CK, Bremner AE **Fractures of the calcaneum. With an atlas illustrating the various types of fracture** J Bone Joint Surg [Br] 1953;35-B: 33–45

Radiology

Lowrie IG, Finlay DB, Brenkel IJ, Gregg PJ **Computerised tomographic assessment of the sub-talar joint in calcaneal fractures** J Bone Joint Surg [Br] 1988;70-B:247–250

Treatment

Soeur R, Remy R **Fractures of the calcaneus with displacement of the thalamic portion** J Bone Joint Surg [Br] 1975;57-B:413–421

Pozo JL, Kirwan EO'G, Jackson AM **The long-term results of conservative management of severely displaced fractures of the calcaneum** J Bone Joint Surg [Br] 1984;66-B:386–390

Stephenson JR **Treatment of displaced intra-articular fractures of the calcaneum using medial and lateral approaches, internal fixation, and early motion** J Bone Joint Surg [Am] 1987;69-A:115–130

Noble J, McQuillan WM **Early posterior sub-talar fusion in the treatment of fractures of the os calcis** J Bone Joint Surg [Br] 1979;61-B:90–93

Essex-Lopresti wrote his classical article in 1952 but his observations on the classification and management of these fractures is still relevant today. **Warrick** shortly afterwards produced an atlas of os calcis fractures giving a description of the various patterns of fractures that can occur.

In 39 fresh fractures of the calcaneus, **Lowrie** showed that the size and disposition of the fracture fragments and the degree of involvement of the posterior facet of the sub-talar joint were more clearly shown by CT scanning than by standard radiography. This technique is recommended for assessment for pre-operative planning. **Soeur** stressed the different types of fracture which may result as a combination of compression and shearing forces. The displaced fragment of the thalamic portion of the calcaneus should be reduced by rotating it and not simply by elevation.

The management of os calcis fractures continues to be controversial and we present three article describing the results of different methods of treatment. **Pozo** reviewed 21 patients with comminuted fractures and severe involvement of the sub-talar joint. He found that with a follow-up of over 14 years three out of four patients had achieved a good result with conservative treatment. It was stressed that the soft tissue injuries were often the cause of long-term disability and these were not affected by reduction of the bony fragments.

Stephenson described an operative technique for reduction and fixation of these fractures; he achieved good results in 21 out of 22 patients with 75% of normal sub-talar movement. Noble in contrast, observed that fractures involving the sub-talar joint frequently caused chronic disability due to subsequent osteoarthritis. Forty-seven cases were reviewed seven years after sub-talar fusion of which 90% had excellent, good or satisfactory results.

One of the difficulties in comparing the treatment of fractures of the os calcis appears to be that the results of contrasting methods are reported as similar.

Mid-Tarsal Injuries

Main BJ, Jowett RL **Injuries of the midtarsal joint** J Bone Joint Surg [Br] 1975; 57-B:89–97

Main classified 71 injuries according to the direction of the deforming force and reviewed the results of treatment, clinically and radiologically. Reduction, open if necessary, with internal fixation is recommended for displaced fractures.

Tarso-Metatarsal Injuries

The Classic

Gisanne W **A dangerous type of fracture of the foot** J Bone Joint Surg [Br] 1951;33-B:535–538

Classification and Treatment

Wiley JJ **The mechanism of tarso-metatarsal joint injuries** J Bone Joint Surg [Br] 1971;53-B:474–482

Hardcastle PH, Reschauer R, Kutscha-Lissberg E, Schoffman W **Injuries to the tarso-metatarsal joint. Incidence, classification and treatment** J Bone Joint Surg [Br] 1982;64-B:349–356

Gisanne emphasised the vascular complications and described the mechanism of damage to the arterial supply to the anterior part of the foot. In **Wiley**'s paper, the anatomy and mechanism of injury is well described based on a study of 20 cases. The paper by **Hardcastle** discussed experience in a multi-centre study with 119 patients treated mostly by closed reduction and K-wire fixation. Whatever the severity of injury, the prognosis depends upon accurate reduction and its maintenance.

Author Index

A page number in bold type indicates a reference by either a single author or the first-named author of a multi-author work.

Abe I 94
Abernethy PJ 56
Ackroyd CE 10
Adams JC **31, 64**
Aharonson Z 17
Ahmed M 9, 103
Ahnqvist S 83
Ainscow DAP 87
Aitken M 15
Akbarnia B **25**
Akermark C 31
Akeson WH 18
Aldgheri R 11
Ali MS **105**
Allan MJ **19**
Allèn PR **95**
Allgower M 6, 7, 9, 36, 47, 98, 102, 105
Alpar EK **24**
Altemeier WA **26**
Alter AJ 73
Andersen E 85
Anderson ID **2**
Anderson JT 9
Anderson LD **42, 71**
Anderson MD 81
Anderson WJ 12
Andersson GBJ 100
Andrews JR 95
Apley AG **100**
Arden GP 97
Ashton F **17**
Ashworth CR 59
Askew L 40
Astrom J **83**
Atasoy E 58
Attenborough CG **37**

Bach AW 103
Bagg RJ 17
Bakalim G 35
Baker SP **2**

Baksi DP **85**
Balkfors B 96
Bannister GC **87**
Barbor P 25
Barnes MJ **107**
Barnes MR 19
Barnes R **84**
Barrett IR 38, 93
Barrington R 85
Barrington TW **92**
Barros D'Sa AAB **18**
Barry HC **14**
Barton NJ 22, **54, 55**
Bassett CAL **8, 103**
Bassett RW **33**
Bauer M **105**
Baxter MP **34**
Beabout EW 53
Beauchamp CG 35, **105**
Beauvill EG 35
Beck G 89
Bedbrook GM **68, 74**
Beertema J 83
Behrens F **10, 102**
Bell MJ **35**
Bellemore MC **38**
Belsky MR **55**
Benke GJ **56**
Benoit RL 37
Bentley GS **84**
Berg E 31
Berg HL 37
Berger A 22, 61
Bergman B 100
Bergman NR **99**
Bergstrathe E 82
Berryman D 70
Beslikas TA 39
Beveridge J 58
Birch R **20, 22, 28**
Birnstingl M **18**
Bjerg-Nielsen A 30
Black J 8
Blair WF 40
Blakemore ME 42, 43

Boales JC 44
Boesen J 15
Boeyens MC 4
Bohlman HH **69**, **74**, 74, 75
Bone LB **3**, **102**
Bonney G **20**
Booy LHD 4
Bora FWM 57
Bose K 40
Bosse MJ 52
Bostman O 4, **35**, 75, **98**
Boyce WJ **83**
Boyd CR **2**
Boyd HB **44**
Boyes JH **58**
Brakenbury PH 42, **43**
Braun RM **21**
Bray T 108
Breedlove RF 74
Bremner AE 110
Brenkel IJ 110
Brighton CT **8**
Broughton RBK 72
Brower TD 12
Brown HG 62
Brown JT 84
Brown PW **50**
Brown RF **36**
Bruce D 100
Brunn F 40
Bryan RS 53, 98
Bucholz RW 3, **76**
Burke DC **70**, **71**
Burke FD 45, **59**, 62, **63**
Burkhalter WE 36, 63
Burny F **7**, **10**
Burstein AH **94**
Burton VW **90**
Bussey R 53
Butler DL **94**, 94
Buxton RA **88**

Cabaud HE **21**
Cadambi A 4
Callahan RA 70
Campbell D **10**
Campbell Reid DA **62**
Canale ST **81**, **88**, **108**
Cannon SR **54**
Carden DG **107**
Carrico CJ 4
Carroll NC 19, 38
Carroll RE **62**
Casteleyn PP **94**
Cattell HS **73**
Catto M **82**
Chacha PB **9**, **103**
Chalmers J **15**, **16**, 46, 107
Champion HJ 2

Chan KM **51**, 73
Chao EY 40
Chapman MW **7**, **9**
Charnley J **6**, **37**, **45**
Chen SC 60
Chisin R 17
Chow YN 51
Christensen J **102**
Christensen P 30
Christiansen C 15
Chuinard RG **63**
Chung SMK 73
Clark CR **71**
Clarke J 85
Claudi B 10
Clawson DK 89
Clay NR 105
Cobbett JR **50**
Cofield RH 33, **98**
Cole WG 90
Coleman DA **40**
Coltart WD **108**
Colwill MR **26**
Conacher WDH 16
Connolly J **18**
Connolly JF 8
Cooke PH **92**
Cooney WP **46**, **53**
Cooper A **82**
Cooperman DR 105
Copeland S **30**
Copes WS 2
Corea JR **42**, 43
Cornish B 72
Crawshaw CV 19
Crock HV **82**
Cross MJ 95
Curtis R 109

Dabezies EJ **90**
Dahlberg E 108
D'Alonzo RT 71
D'Ambrosia RD 63, 80, 90
Dameron TB 95
Dandy DJ **94**, 95, **96**
Daruwalla JS 9, 103
Das SK **62**
Davis T 9
Day L 35
Day LJ 8
De Bastiani G **11**
De Dombal FT 2
De Graff AC 4
de Oliveira JC **7**
De Silva RDD 28
De Souza LJ **105**
Dean AE 61
Debruyn PF 10
DeLee JC **109**

Deliyannis SN **42**
Denham RA 95
Denis F **68**
Dennis BA 70
Devas MB **16, 86**
Dias JJ **30, 46**
Dick HM 12
Dickson RA 52
Dickson WA 50
Dobyns JH 46, 53
Dommisse GF 4
Dooley BJ **52**
Dove J **14**
Dowd GSE 54
Doyle JR 61
Drake D 35
Dray GJ **56**
Dreyfuss UY **64**
Duckworth T 105
Duke JH 2
Duncan A 77
Dussault RG 72

Eadie DGA **18**
Eaton RG 55, 56
Edeiken-Monroe B 69
Edmondson RS **26**
Edvardsen P **90**
Effendi B **72**
Ejeskar A **58**
Ellis H **101**
Ellis J **47**, 107
Ellison LH 4
Enis JE 12
Epstein HC **80**, 81
Esah M 41
Esser MP **87**
Essex-Lopresti P **109**
Esterhai JL 8
Evans DK **70**, 72
Evans DM **50**
Evans EM **44, 86**
Evans GA **106, 107**
Evarts CM 85

Fidler MW **13**
Fielding JW **73**
Filtzer DL 73
Finlay DB 110
Fischer RP **2**
Fisher TR **22**
Fisher WE 52
Fisk GR **53**
Fitzgerald B 41
Fitton JM 107
Fleming LL 102
Fletcher I 61
Flynn JC **37**
Flynn TC 2

Fordyce AJW 90
Foster RJ **54**
Fowles JV 39
Fragiadakis EG 56, 61
Franklin A **85**
Fraser RD **91, 104**
Fredrickson BE 74
Freedlander E **50**
Frenyo AD 107
Frenyo SD 106
Friedenberg ZB 8
Friedlaender GE **7**
Fullen WD 26
Fuller DJ **44, 47**
Fyfe IS **42**

Gaines RW **74**
Gainor BJ 59
Galasko CSB **12**
Galey JP 45
Gallagher JC **82**
Gallannaugh SC 85
Galleno H **25**
Galvin EG 35
Ganz R 31
Garden RS **84**, 84
Gardner DL 16
Garetto LP 18
Gartsman GM **42**
Gaston SR 8, 103
Gelberman RH 52
George J 107
Gerber C **31**
Gertzbein SD **74**
Getty CJM 81
Gibson AGF 87
Giladi M 17
Gimbrere JSF 4
Gingras MB **85**
Gisanne W **111**
Glass KD **63**
Godfrey AM **64**
Goldberg V 99
Goldstein A **77**
Goldstein J 77
Goletz TH 73
Goodman MA **14**
Goris RJA **4**
Gossling HR **4**, 23
Graham HK 37
Grant JP **4**
Grantham SA 92
Green DP 30, **53**
Green SA **11**
Gregg PJ 30, 46, 110
Griffiths DL **14**
Gristina AG 12
Grob D **108**
Grood ES **94**, 94

Grosse A 89
Grundy DJ **68, 70**
Gruninger RP 9
Gruss JS 103
Gurd AR **4**
Gustilo RB **9**, 43, 105

Habermann ER **12**
Hadden WA **42**
Haddon W Jr 2
Hakkinen S 4
Hall G **87**
Hamblen DL **70**
Hampson WGJ **99**
Handelberg F 94
Hansen ST 89, 91, 103
Hansen TR Jr 104
Hardcastle P 107
Hardcastle PH **111**
Hardy AE **89**, 107
Hargens AR 18
Harper D 61
Harrington KD **12, 13**
Harris JH **69**
Harris WR 24
Harrison SH **50**
Hart L 70
Harvey JP 93, 97
Harvey L 83
Harviel JD **2**
Hassman GC **40**
Hastings H 54
Haw CS 53
Hawkins RJ **33**, 73
Hayken GD 57
Hegedus V 15
Heim U **55, 104**
Helal B **60, 91**
Heller FG 105
Hendricks P 81
Henning CE 95
Henry AK **35, 43**
Herbert TJ **52**
Herberts P 31
Herkowitz HN **72**
Herold HZ 40
Heyse-Moore GH **87**
Heywood AWB **98**
Heyworth J **3**
Hidaka S **43**
Hill P 99
Hirsh DM 12
Ho KC 15
Hobbs CJ **25**
Hoffman E 2
Holden CEA **19, 38, 44**
Holdsworth BJ **42**, 42
Holdsworth FW **76**
Holdsworth Sir F **68**

Holstein A **35**
Holzach P 36
Honner R **61**
Hooper G **60**
Horn G 92
Hosking DJ 83
Hovelius L **31**
Hudson LD 4
Hughes AD 17
Hughes JL **105**
Hughes SPF 28
Hughston JC **95, 99**
Hull D 25
Hungerford DS 23
Hunter GA **85**, 87, 91, 104
Hvass I 85

Innes AR 45
Insall JN **97, 99**
Ions GK **83**
Ireland J **94**
Irving M 2
Iwegbu G 60

Jabaley M **21**
Jackson AM 110
Jackson IT 50
Jackson JP **94**
Jackson RW **94**, 95
Jakob R **39**
James ETR **87, 103**
James JIP **50, 55**
Jameson-Evans DC 87
Jaroma H 4
Jarvinen M 96
Jeffery CC **39, 41**
Jenkins NH **46**
Jenning JJ 36
Jenson GF **15**
Jenson J 94
Jenson JS **83, 86**
Johansen KH 103
Johansson JE 92
Johnson KD **4**, 102
Johnson RM **70**
Johnson SR 46
Johnston JO 12
Jolly BL 95
Jones DG 46
Jones DHA 87
Jones ERL **41**
Jones JM 46
Jonsson B 83
Jonsson K 105
Jorgen G 102
Jowett RL 111
Juett DA 89
Jupiter JB **36**

Kaltas D-S **17, 86**
Kannus P **96**
Karadimas J **32**
Karlstrom G 6
Kashtan H 17
Kassab JY 87
Kassab MT 39
Katz MM **23**
Kaufman HD **63**
Keene JS **73**
Kellam J 91
Kellam JK 35
Kelly EG 70
Kelly FB 108
Kelly PJ **7**
Kempf I **89**
Kempson GF 10
Kessel L 30
Kinman PB 35, 100
Kinmonth MH **50**
Kirkpatrick J 25
Kirwan EO'G 110
Kiviluoto O 4, 98
Kleinert HE **58**, 58, 64
Klenerman L **35**
Kline DG **21**
Knight PN 61
Kopaniky DR 69
Korner L 31, 100
Kostuik JP **70, 75**
Krajbich JI 37
Krieg JK 29, 35
Krishnamoorthy S **40**
Krugmire RB 18
Kuczynski K **56**
Kuner EH 105
Kuntscher G **89**
Kutscha-Lissberg E 111
Kutz JE **55**, 58

Lam SF 88
Lamb DW 53, **54, 56, 58**, 61, **73**
Lane JM **12, 15, 83**
Lang-Stevenson A **81**
Lange RH **103**
Langenskiold A **24**
Lansinger O **100**
Laros GS **87**, 105
Larson E **30**
Latta LL 92, 100
Laurin CA 72
Lauritzen J 94
Leddy JE **63**
Leffert RD **28, 32, 34**
Leslie IJ **52**
Leslie JT **32**
Letournel E **80**
Letts M **44**
Leung PC 51, **88**

Lewis J **74**
Lilleas F 74
Linde F **85**
Lindeque BGP **4**
Linscheid RL 46, **53**, 53
Lister GD **50, 58**, 64
Locht R 44
Lombardo SJ **93**
London PS **52**
Long WB 2
Lowell JD 80
Lowell M 81
Lowrie IG **110**
Lubicky JP 74
Lundberg B 31
Lunn P 107

Ma GFY 51
McAfee PC **74**
McBroom RJ 92, 100
McCarroll HR 21, 61
McCartney WH 17
McCoy GF 37
McCullough CJ 44
McDaniel WJ **95**
MacEachern AG 87
McGinnis GH 96
McGraw RW **71**
McGregor IA 50
McGrouther DA 50
Mack GR **52**
Mackay I **41**
McKibbin B **6, 23**, 74
MacLaren A 46
McLaren CAN 105
McLaughlin HL **32, 33**
MacLeod AM 62
MacMichael D 74
McMullen H 107
McMurtry RY 35, **76**
McQueen MM **46**
McQuillan WM 110
McSweeney T 72
Madsen F 85
Mahoney M 9
Main BJ **111**
Mankin HJ **16**
Mann RJ 63
Manugian AH 81
Marar BC 69, **71**
Margulies JY 17
Marsh D **22**
Marshall RW **28**
Massiah KA 76
Mast JW 105
Matev I **60**
Matsen FA **18**
Matta JM **81**
Matter M 9

Matthews JG 37
Matthews P **57**
Mattingly DA 35
Maudsley RH 26
Mears A 58
Meggitt BF 88, **89**
Meissl G 22, 61
Melone CP **46**
Melton LJ 15, 82
Meyer S **7**, 37
Meyer TJ 105
Meyers MH **97**
Middleton RWD 38
Mikic ZD **40**, **45**
Milford L **60**, **61**
Milgrom C **17**
Miller JH 41
Miller PW 2
Millesi H **20**, **22**, **61**
Mintowt-Czyz WJ 46
Mitchell JP **77**
Mitchell SN 8, 103
Moberg E **21**
Monahan PRW **76**
Mooney V **10**
Moore JF 87
Morgan RG 36
Morrey BF **40**
Morrison WA **62**
Moschi A 95
Moss JG **59**
Mossad MM 42
Moulton A 80
Mouradian WH 13
Mouritsen P 94
Mubarak SJ **18**, **19**, 38
Mueller J 37
Mulfinger GL **108**
Muller ME **6**, **7**, **47**, **98**
Mulligan PJ **55**
Munson G 74
Murphy G 90
Murray JF 23, **62**
Mutz SB 21
Myllynen P 75

Narakas A **28**
Neer CS **29**, **33**, **34**, 40, **92**
Neff U 36
Newman JH **41**, 92
Nicholson JT 73
Nicoll EA **7**, **74**, **84**, 84, **101**
Niebauer JJ 21, 61
Nielsen AB **44**
Nilsson B 96, 105
Nirhamo J 98
Nistor L **107**
Nobel W **32**
Noble J **17**, 53, 107, **110**

Norris R 90
Norris SH **71**, 105
Northmore-Ball MD **95**
Noyes FR 94, **96**
Nusynowitz ML 17

O'Brien BM 62
O'Brien ET 53
O'Connor BT 10, 105
Ogden JA **24**, **100**
Olerud S **6**
Omer GE **21**, **22**
O'Neill B 2
Opdecam P 94
Oppenheim WL 25
Osmond-Clarke H **31**
Osterman AL **57**
Otis JC 42
Owen CA 18
Owen JR 70
Owen R 24

Paavilainen T 4
Pahud B **6**
Pallesen R 85
Panetta T 77
Panjabi MM 72
Pankovich AM **105**
Panting AL **53**
Papavasiliou VA **39**
Park WI 42
Park WM 72
Patel D 31
Patiala A 35
Pawley E 83
Payan J **22**
Peltier LF **4**
Pennal GF **76**
Pepe PE **4**
Peterson L **108**
Pfeiffer KM 55, 104
Phillips JG 35
Phillips T 77
Pho RWH **9**
Piggot J **37**
Pirone AM **37**
Plewes LW **23**
Pollen AG **54**, **63**
Pollock FH **35**
Pomeroy DL 35
Poplawski ZJ **23**
Poppen NK **61**
Potkin RT 4
Potts H 17
Pozo JL **110**
Prather JL **17**
Pringle RG **62**
Pritchard DJ 12
Pritchett JW **35**

Pulvertaft RG **57**
Pussey RJ 96

Radin EL 36, **40**
Raess DH 2
Raggi RP **51**
Rainey HA 97
Ramamurthy S **51**
Rang M **24**, **37**, **39**, 39, **43**, **90**, 90, **93**
Ransford AO **28**
Rashkoff ES **63**
Rasquin C 7
Ratliff AHC **62**, **88**
Reckling FW **45**, **103**
Remy R 110
Rentis G 32
Renzibrivio L 11
Reschauer R 42, 111
Reus DH 4
Reynolds DA **24**
Reynolds DS **90**
Richards HJ 57, **58**
Richardson RA 30
Rickard TA 59
Riggs BL **15**, 82
Riseborough EH **36**
Riseborough EJ 40, **93**
Riska EB **4**, **75**
Rittmann WW **9**
Roberton DM **25**
Robinson AR 61
Rockwood CA **30**
Rodhey WG 21
Rokkanen P 35
Romanis B 108
Roper BA **89**
Rorabeck CH **19**
Rosen H **7**
Rosen MJ 29
Rosendahl S 102
Rothman RH 72
Rouholamin E 105
Rowe CR **29**, **31**, **32**, **80**
Rowley DI **105**
Roy D 72
Ruedi TP **35**, **43**, **102**, **105**
Ruff ME 55
Rusch RM 71
Russell J 68
Ryan TJ 32
Ryle DP 80

Sach R 12
Sackett JF 73
Sage FP 7
Saibil E 76
Salter RB **24**
Salvati E 99
Salvatore JE **30**

Sandberg R **96**
Sarmiento AA **35**, **92**, **100**, **101**
Satku K 9
Scalea T 77
Schatzker J **10**, **92**, 92, **100**
Scheker L 50
Schibli M 9
Schmitt RH 35
Schneider R 6, 7, 47, 98
Schoeman HS 4
Schoffman W 111
Schoots FJ 4
Schulmpf R 35, 43
Schutzer SF **23**
Sclafani SJA 77
Scott GA **95**
Scott JC **98**
Scott JE **61**
Scott JM 54
Scott PJ 16
Scougall JS 38
Sculco TP 12, 42
Searls K 102
Seddon HJ **19**, 34
Seddon Sir HJ **20**, **28**, 28, **32**, **38**
Sedel L **28**
Sefton GK **107**
Seggl W 42
Seibert GB 4
Semple C **50**
Sevitt S **4**
Shaftan G 77
Shapiro F 93
Shelton ML 92
Shelton WR **7**
Sherk HH **73**
Shmueli G **40**
Shoji H 90
Shouse L 105
Shurr D 40
Sikorski JM **85**
Silver JR **68**
Sim FH **12**, 12
Simms MH **18**
Simonsen O 44, **94**
Simpson LA 108
Singer M 64
Sisk TD 42
Skevis X 91
Slaney G 17
Smith JD 89
Smith R **12**, **14**, **15**, **16**
Smith RJ **57**
Sneddon J 64
Snowdy HA 17
Soeur R **110**
Solomon L **82**
Souter WA **60**
Southmayd WW 31

Spiegel PG **105**
Springfield DS **12**
Stableforth PG **34**
Stack HG **59**
Stark HH 58, **59**
Stauffer ES **69, 70, 74**
Stein M 17
Steinberg R 17
Steingold RF 30, 59
Stenner B **56, 57**
Stephenson JR **110**
Stern PJ **35**
Stern RE 12
Stevens J 83
Stewart HD **45**
Stewens A 83
Stirling AJ 19
Stoker DJ 94
Stromqvist B **85**
Sugi M **90**
Suntay WJ 94
Sussman S 25
Swain A 68
Swan AV 95
Swiontkowski MC **91**
Syversen SM 90
Szabo RM 46

Taleisnik J **53**
Taylor AR **97**
Taylor RG 76
Tesfayohannes B 30
Thal ER **2**
Thexton PW 105
Thomas FB **47**
Thomas TL **88**
Tile M 10, 74, **76, 77, 80, 81, 104, 105, 108**
Tipton WW **80**
Tolo VT 37
Tolson MA 2
Tooms RE 42
Torg JS 25
Trafton PG 35
Transbol I 15
Trickey EL 94, **96**
Trueta J 108
Trunkey DD **2**
Tubiana R **58**

Upadhyay SS **80**
Urbaniak JR **21**
Uribe JW 36

Vainionpaa S 35
Vajara R 9
Van Niekerk JLM 4
Varian JPW **58, 60**
Varouchas G 32
Vasey H 6

Veith RG **91, 104**
Velazco A **102**
Verdan CE **57**
Vessey MP 83
Vigorita VJ 15, 83
Vlok AL 4
von Bonsdorff H 4
Von Hochstetter AHC 35, 43
Vukadinovic SV 40

Waddell J 92
Waddell JB **91**, 104
Wallace WA 34
Walsh WM 99
Warrick CK **110**
Waters CH 103
Watt I 71
Webb JK **72**, 102
Weber BG **23**, 108
Weber H 105
Weber SC **46**
Weigelt JA **4**
Weiland AJ 7, **9, 37**
Weins J 44
Westlin N 96
White AA 71, **72**
Whitesides TE 102
Whiteway DW 38
Wiley AM 23
Wiley JJ 34, **45, 111**
Wilkinson J **98**
Willenegger H 6, 7, 47, 98, 105
Williams DH 54
Williams PF 99
Wilppula E 35
Wilson JN **11**
Wilson RI 4
Wilton TJ **83**
Winquist RA 18, **89**, 91, 104
Wong KP 40
Woodford M 2
Worlock P **37**
Wray CC 46
Wredmark T 31
Wynn Parry CB **20, 28, 61, 65**

Yablon IG **105**
Yates DW 3
Young TB **34**
Yu E 52
Yuan HA 74, 75

Zagorski JB **36**
Zarins B 32
Zemel NP 59
Zenni EJ **29**, 35
Zickel RE **13, 89**
Ziv I **90**
Zolan S 12

Subject Index

Acetabulum, fractures 77, 80–1
Achilles tendon rupture 107–8
Acromioclavicular joint 30–1
Adult respiratory distress syndrome 4
Anaesthesia, hand surgery 51
Ankle, lateral ligament injury 106–7
Ankle fractures 104–6
    classification 104
    comparison of operative and conservative
        treatment 105
    evaluation of 105
    in the elderly 105
    long-term follow-up 105
    surgical treatment 105
    tri-plane fractures 105
Arterial injuries 17, 18
Atlanto-axial arthodesis 71
Avascular necrosis 85
Aviator's astragalus 108

Bankart procedure 31
Battered child syndrome 25
Bennett's fracture 54
Bladder injury 77–8
Blood transfusion 4
Bone grafts
    basic science 7
    historical 7
    infection 7
    non-union 7
    operative technique 7
    treatment 7
    vascularised 9
Boutonnière deformity 60
Brachial plexus injuries 28–9
Bristow–Latarjet procedure 31

Calcaneum fractures 109–11
Carpal dislocations 53
Carpal instability 53–4
Cervical dislocations 70
Cervical instability 72
Cervical orthoses 70

Cervical spine
    fractures 13
    injuries 69–71
        hyperextension 71
        in children 73
Cervicothoracic junction dislocations 70
Child abuse 25
Clavicle
    fractures 29–30
    non-union 29
Colles' fracture 45–7
Compartment syndromes 18–19
Cubitus varus 38

Dens fracture 71
Digital nerve 61
Digits
    dislocation and ligament injuries 56–7
    replantation 64–5
Distal humerus
    epiphyseal injuries 39
    fractures 36
Dorso-lumbar spine 74

Elbow dislocation 40
Electrical stimulation 8
Electromyography 22
Ellis plate operation 47
Epineurial nerve suture 21
Epiphyseal injuries, distal humerus 39
Epiphyseal plate 24
Epiphysis 23
Extensor pollicis longus tendon 60

Fascicular nerve suture 21
Fat embolism 4
Femoral head necrosis 85
Femoral neck fractures 16, 82, 84–6
in children 88
Femoral shaft fractures 6, 88–9
    in children 90–1
Femur

associated injuries 91
ipsi-lateral fractures 104
metastatic disease 12
subcapital fractures 84–5
sub-trochanteric region 13
supracondylar fractures
in adult 92–3
in children 93
Finger injuries 56
Finger tip injuries and amputations 61–3
Foot, sub-talar dislocation 109
Forearm fractures 43
in children 44
Fractures
early stabilisation 4
external fixation 10–11
healing 23
infection 9
inter-trochanteric 86–7
intercondylar 36
internal fixation 4, 6
long bone 6, 15
management of 3
mid-clavicular 29
non-union 7
open 9–10
pathological 11–17
post-menopausal spinal 15
repair 6
septic non-union 11
stress 16–17, 86
supracondylar 37, 92–3
*see also under named fractures and specific
organs*

Galeazzi fracture 45
Gas gangrene 26
Grease gun injuries 63
Growth plate 24

Halo immobilisation 70
Hand
fractures 17, 54–6
human bite infections 63–4
infections 63
injury 50
nerve injuries 60–1
rehabilitation 28, 65
replantation 64–5
sensibility 21
surgery, anaesthesia 51
Hangman's fracture 72
Harrington instrumentation 74–5
High pressure injection injuries 63
Hip dislocation 80–1
Hip fractures
bi-articular prosthesis 85

in children 88
in rheumatoid arthritis 85
in the elderly 82
Hip replacement
complicating total 92
endoprosthetic 12
Humeral condyle fractures 39
Humeral shaft fractures 35–6
Humerus
intercondylar fractures 36
supracondylar fractures 37

Infections
bone grafts 7
hand 63
tendon sheath 63
Infraclavicular brachial plexus injuries 32
Injuries
assessment of 2
closed 4
deaths from 2
helicopter response to 2
management of 2, 3
multiple 4
musculo-skeletal 4, 24
severity score 2
Inter-trochanteric fractures 86–7
Intramedullary nailing 89

Knee
arthrography 94
arthroscopy 94
chronic instability 97
dislocations 97
ligament injuries 95–7
soft tissue injuries 94–7

Laminectomy 69
Leg
double-incision fasciotomy 18
injuries 19
Ligament injuries, knee 95–7
Long bones
fractures 6, 15
growth changes in 24
Lower limb
metastases 12
Volkmann's ischaemia 19

Malgaigne fracture-dislocation of the pelvis 76
Malignant disease 12–13
Malleolar fractures 104
Mallet finger 59
Mechanical ventilation 4
Medial epicondyle injury 39

Median nerve 61
Meniscus, injuries of 95
Meniscectomy 95
Metacarpal fractures 54
Midtarsal joint injuries 111
Monteggia fracture 44
Muscular skeletal injuries, in children 24
Musculo-skeletal injuries 4
  in children 24
Myelomatosis 14

Nerve grafting 22
Nerve injuries, hand 60–1
Neuroma, evaluation 21
Nicoll-graft treatment 7
Nutrition 4

Odontoid fractures 71
Olecranon fractures 42
Osteomalacia 16, 83
Osteomyelitis 7
Osteoporosis 15, 83
Osteosynthesis 4

Paediatric trauma 23–6
Paget's disease of bone 14
Papineau technique 7
Paraplegia 68, 74
Partial physeal arrest 24
Patella
  dislocations 98–9
  fractures 98
Pelvis, fractures 76–8
Perichondrial ring 24
Perineal nerve repair 21
Peripheral nerve disorders 28
Peripheral nerve injuries 20–2
Phalangeal fractures 55
Pipkin fracture-dislocation of the hip 81
Plasma cell tumours 14
Post-traumatic ischaemia 18
Proximal humeral fractures 33–4
Pseudarthroses 7
Putti-Platt operation 31

Radial head fractures 40
  in children 41
Radial neck fractures, in children 41
Radial shaft fractures 42–3
  in children 43
Reflex sympathetic dystrophy 23
Remodelling 24
Renal osteodystrophy 16
Replantation 64–5
Respiratory failure 4

Rheumatoid arthritis, hip fracture in 85
Rickets 16
Ring of the axis fractures 72
Road accidents 2
Rotator cuff tears 33

Scaphoid fractures 52
Sensation 20
Sensibility, hand 21
Shock, recognition and treatment 2
Shoulder joint dislocation 31–3
Skeletal disorders 12
Skeletal metastases 12
Skull fracture 25
Skull traction 70
Smith's fracture 47
Soft tissue injuries, knee 94–7
Spinal cord deficiency 69
Spinal cord injuries 68–9
Spinal fractures, dislocations and fracture-
    dislocations 68
Spinal injuries
  classification and mechanisms of 68
  hyperextension 71
  see also Cervical spine injuries; Dorso-lumbar
    spine;
    Thoracolumbar spine
Spinal instability 68
Spinal metastases 13
Spinal trauma 68
Sternoclavicular joint 30
Stress fractures 16–17, 86
Subcapital fractures 84
Subscapularis tendon 32
Sudeck's atrophy 23

Talus fracture 108–9
Tarso-metatarsal injuries 111
Tendon injuries
  extensor 59–60
  flexor 57–9
Tendon sheaths, infection 63
Tendons, subscapularis 32
Tetanus 26
Tetraplegia 68, 73
Thoracolumbar spine injuries 74–6
Thumb
  amputations 62
  metacarpophalangeal joint 56–7
  reconstruction 62
Tibia
  associated injuries 91
  ipsi-lateral fractures 104
  management of fractures 104
  plateau fractures 100
  shaft fractures 101–4
Tibiofibular joint dislocation 100

Trauma
  care evaluation 2
  multiple 3, 4
  nutrition 4
TRISS method 2

Ulna shaft fractures 42–3
  in children 43
Ulnar nerve 61
Upper limb
  metastases 12
  paralysis 73
Urethra injury 77–8
Urinary tract trauma 77

Vascular injuries 17–20
Vertebral fractures 74
Volkmann's contracture 19–20, 38, 44

Wick catheter 18
Wrist
  fractures 53
  septic arthritis 63